Did You Hear That?

Help for Children Who Hear Voices

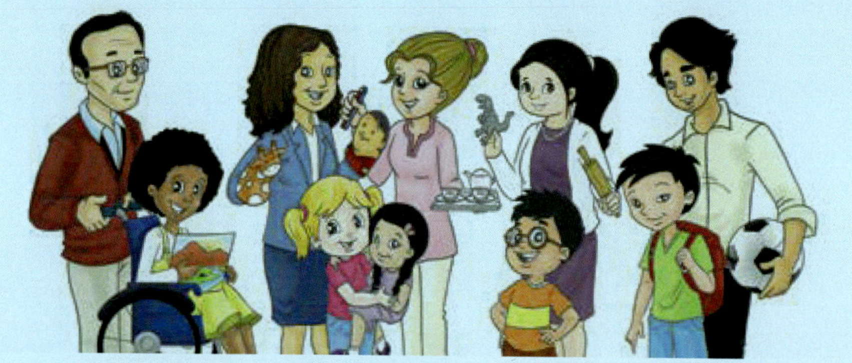

Did You Hear That?

Help for Children Who Hear Voices

Written by

Seetha Subbiah, MA, PsyD

Clinical Psychologist

Illustrated by

Abi Das

Published by

WS Education, an imprint of
World Scientific Publishing Co. Pte. Ltd.
5 Toh Tuck Link, Singapore 596224
USA office: 27 Warren Street, Suite 401-402, Hackensack, NJ 07601
UK office: 57 Shelton Street, Covent Garden, London WC2H 9HE

British Library Cataloguing-in-Publication Data
A catalogue record for this book is available from the British Library.

DID YOU HEAR THAT?
Help for Children Who Hear Voices

ISBN 978-981-3144-14-9
ISBN 978-981-3144-15-6 (pbk)

Printed in Singapore

Preface

Until 2006, there was very limited research done in the area of auditory and visual hallucinations among children. In my clinical work with child clients who heard voices, it was evident that the root cause for the phenomenon was not always organic in nature and did not always require pharmacotherapy. Also evident was the emotional turmoil and psychological suffering associated with the phenomenon. Child clients struggled to verbalize their experiences and these symptoms interfered with their optimal functioning. Unfortunately, appropriate treatment tools for this population were scarce at the time. In order to help these kids, I wrote an early version of this book in 2006.

In its unillustrated, Microsoft Word format, it was used as a treatment tool for child clients and training resource for interns and practicum students in the intensive outpatient program at EMQ Families First, a community mental health service provider in California. After two years, the feedback from therapists who used the book with child clients was very positive. Over the next few years I continued to fine-tune it to make it a dynamic and informative tool to help mental health providers, such as psychologists, psychiatrists, psychotherapists, counselors and clinical social workers in their work with child clients.

Written in very simple terms, child clients will find it easy to understand. Clinicians can read this book to younger clients while older ones can read it themselves. Because of the way the book is structured, both groups have the option of pacing themselves through the book by choosing to read on or skip parts.

Designed as a therapeutic storybook, it can be included as part of clinicians' permanent book collection in their office so child clients can access it at any time to read, if interested. Therapists with a more directive style can actively introduce this book to clients as desired. Hence, professionals that subscribe to either a non-directive or directive style of therapy would find this book useful in their work with clients.

In summary, this book can assist to:

- Introduce the condition of auditory and visual hallucinations into the treatment room in a non-threatening manner
- Help child clients to express their feelings and struggles associated with hallucinatory experiences
- Assist child clients to explore the specificities of their hallucinatory experiences and possible root causes
- Normalize the experience for child clients by helping them realize that other children experience this phenomenon
- Support child clients as they explore options and strategies to cope with the phenomenon
- Elicit child clients' preferences regarding what role they would like voices to play in their lives
- Help child clients find ways to share, express and communicate their struggles with voices to trusted adults
- Elicit whether a child client's visual and auditory experiences could indicate an organic condition that may need further assessment, diagnosis and treatment in early adulthood
- Help the child client embrace rather than fear the phenomenon, especially when the condition may be organic in nature
- Provide perspective and understanding through education to parents, siblings, and extended family members, as well as professionals who may encounter children who experience this phenomenon, such as teachers, medical doctors, speech therapists, occupational therapists, other healthcare professionals, probation officers, and lawyers.

My personal hope for this multidimensional book is for it to reach and assist as many children as possible who may be suffering in silence or in isolation. By reducing the incidence of false positive diagnoses of psychosis in children, the unnecessary use of anti-psychotic medication can be reduced and instead, appropriate clinical treatment can be rendered to help them understand, accept, master and cope with their voices. It is hoped that this book will be a gentle, empathic, and compassionate companion and guide to children in their journey to living effective and successful lives with voices.

CONTENT

Chapter One

The One-Legged Pirate

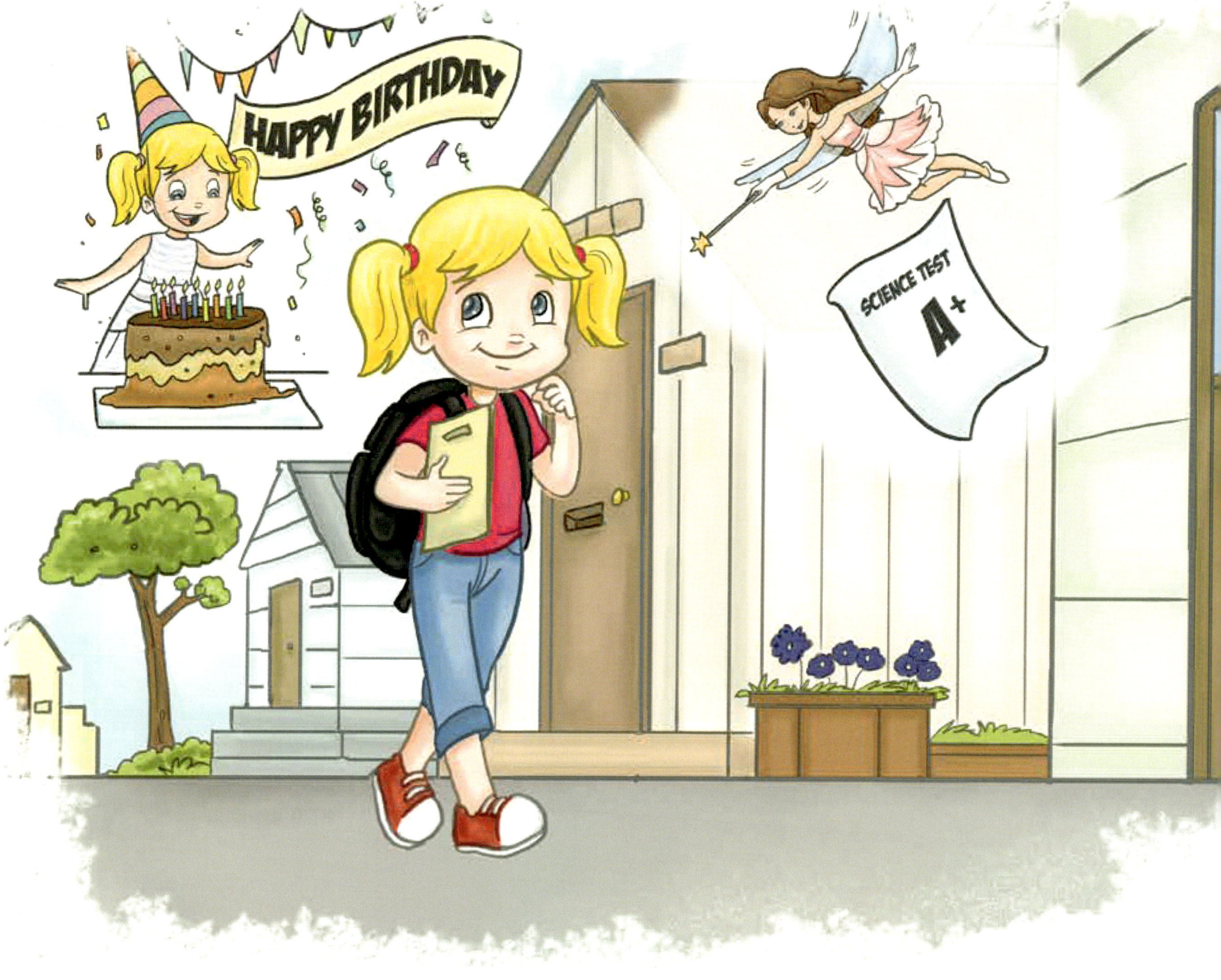
HAPPY BIRTHDAY
SCIENCE TEST
A+

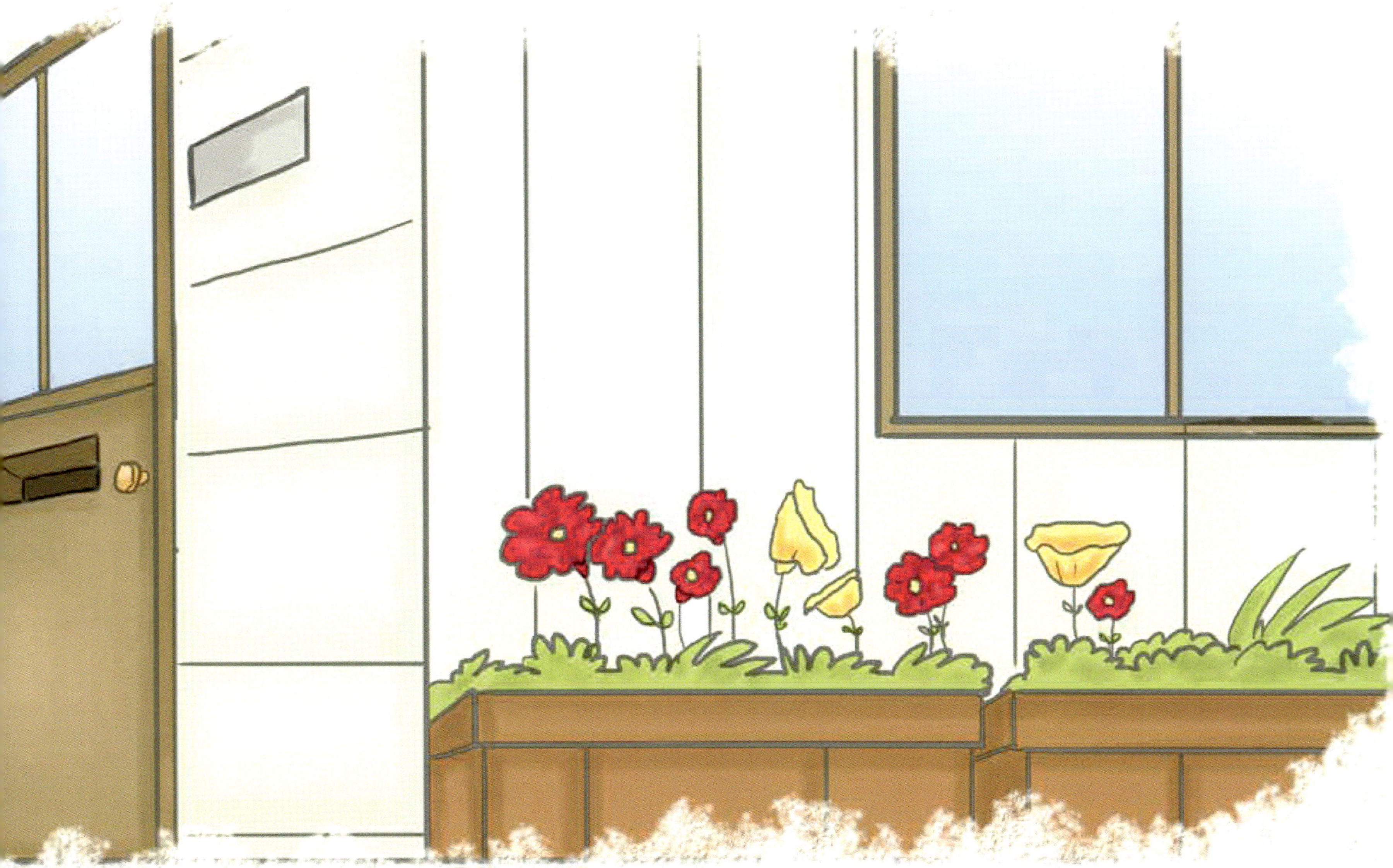

Turning 9 years old two days ago was going to change my life. Things were going to be different, including my science grade. Well, at least I hoped so.

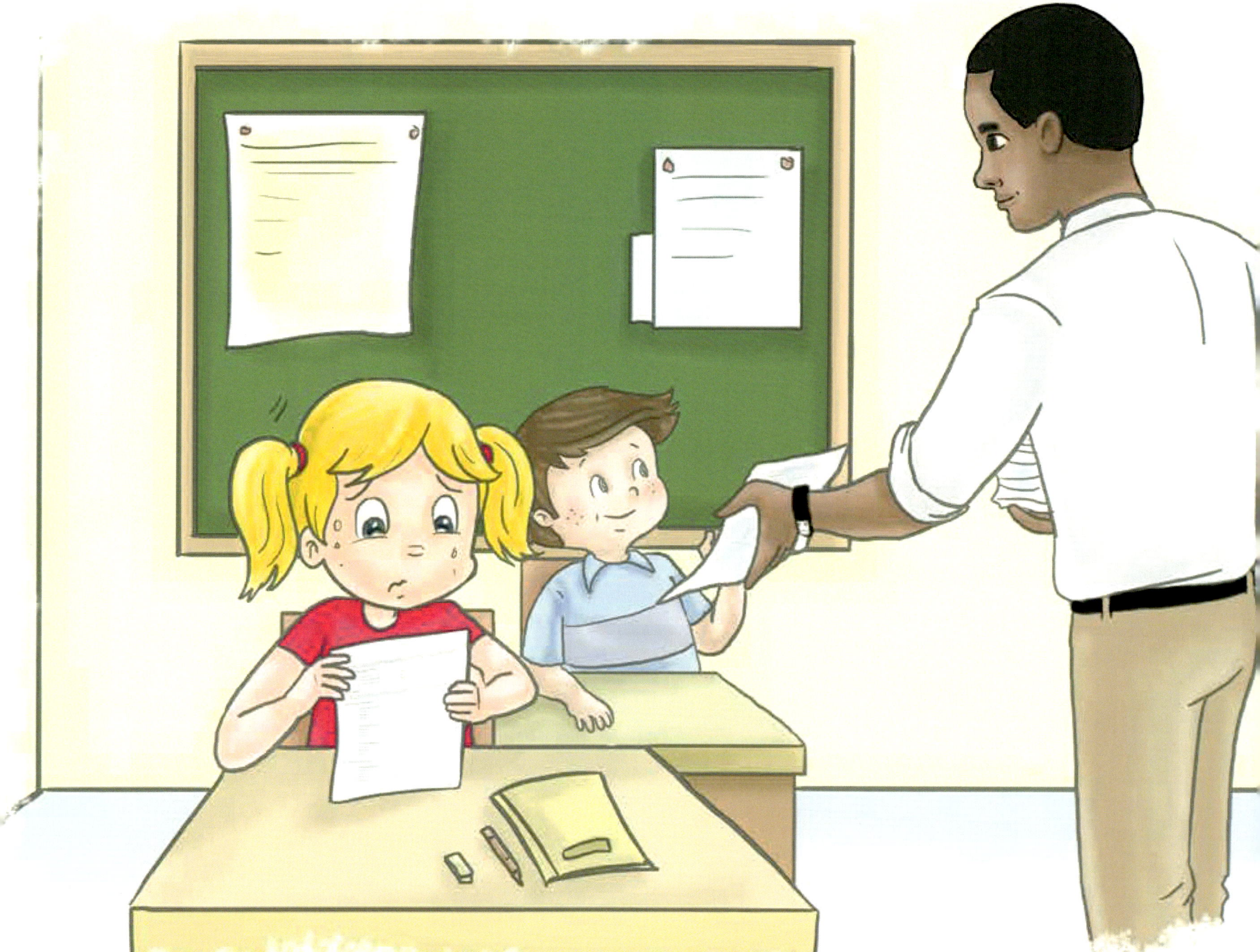

I was sitting at my desk at school when my teacher, Mr Jones, handed me my science test sheet.

I turned it over and barely finished reading the first question when that thing happened again!

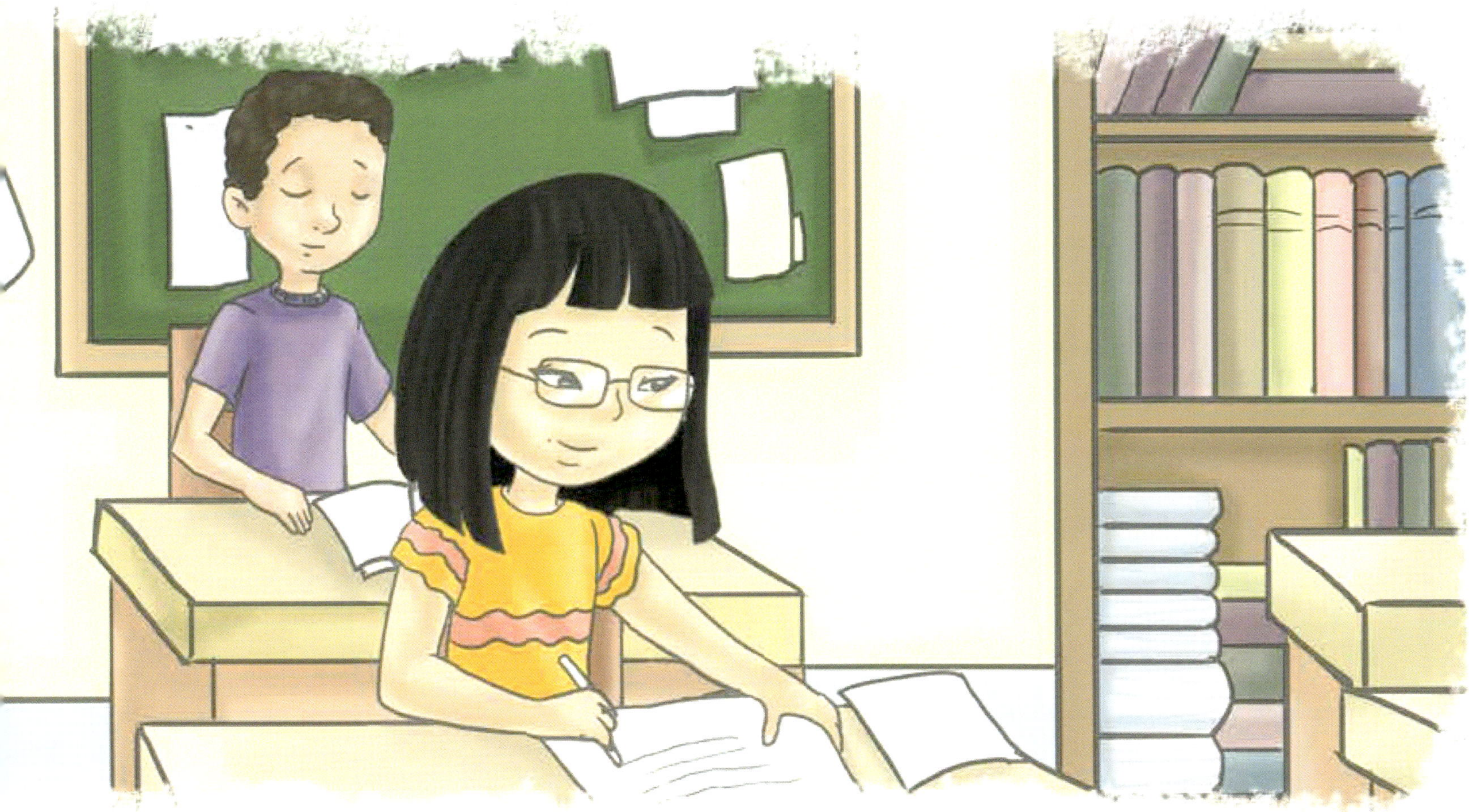

I couldn't believe it. That dreadful thing happened again!

I thought to myself, "I'm so weird".

The horrible one-legged pirate's voice kept saying things.

"Pick answer A. No, no, no pick C! B, B, answer B is the right one, you numbskull!"

The one-legged pirate's voice chattered on and on and on in my head.

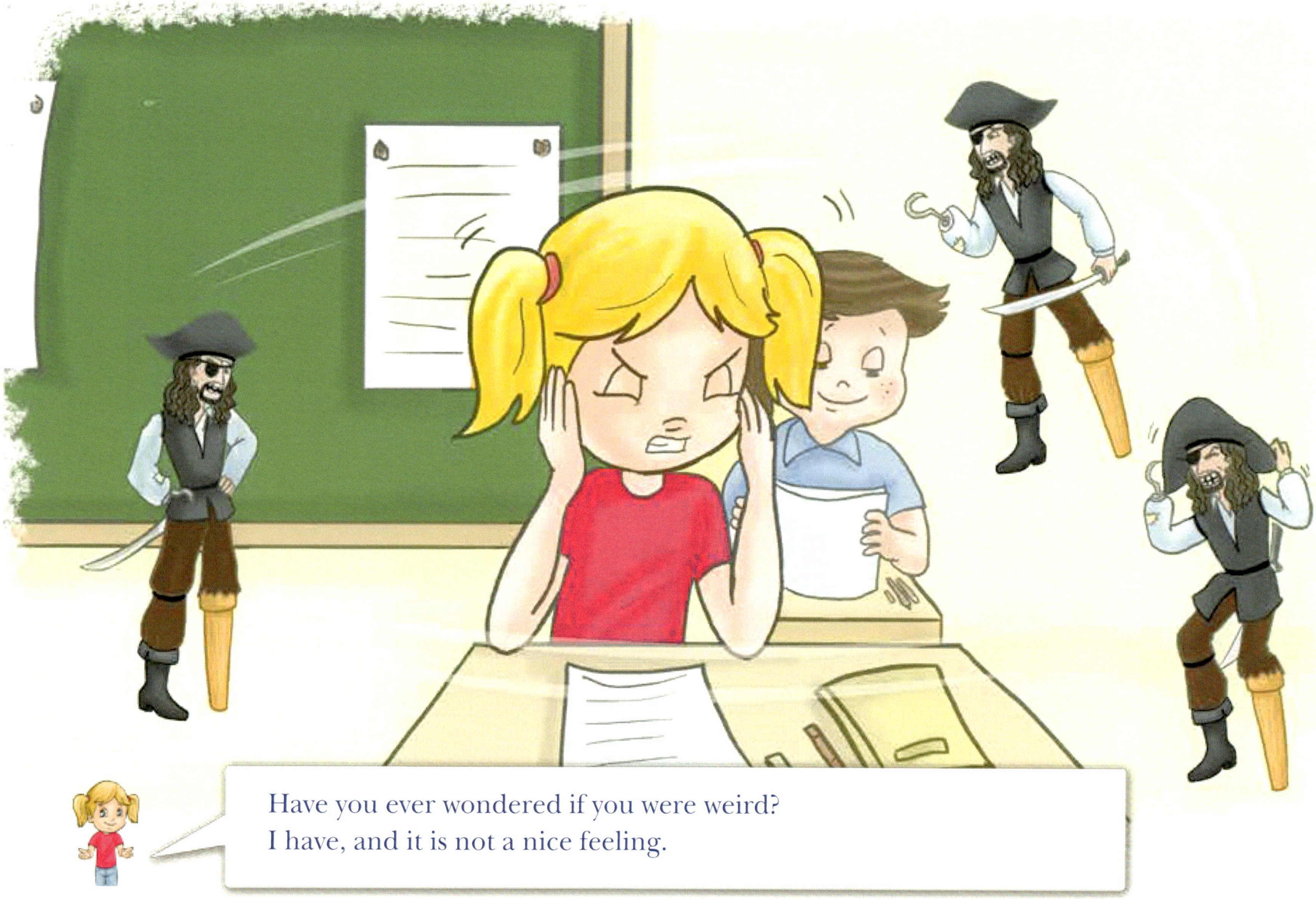
Have you ever wondered if you were weird?
I have, and it is not a nice feeling.

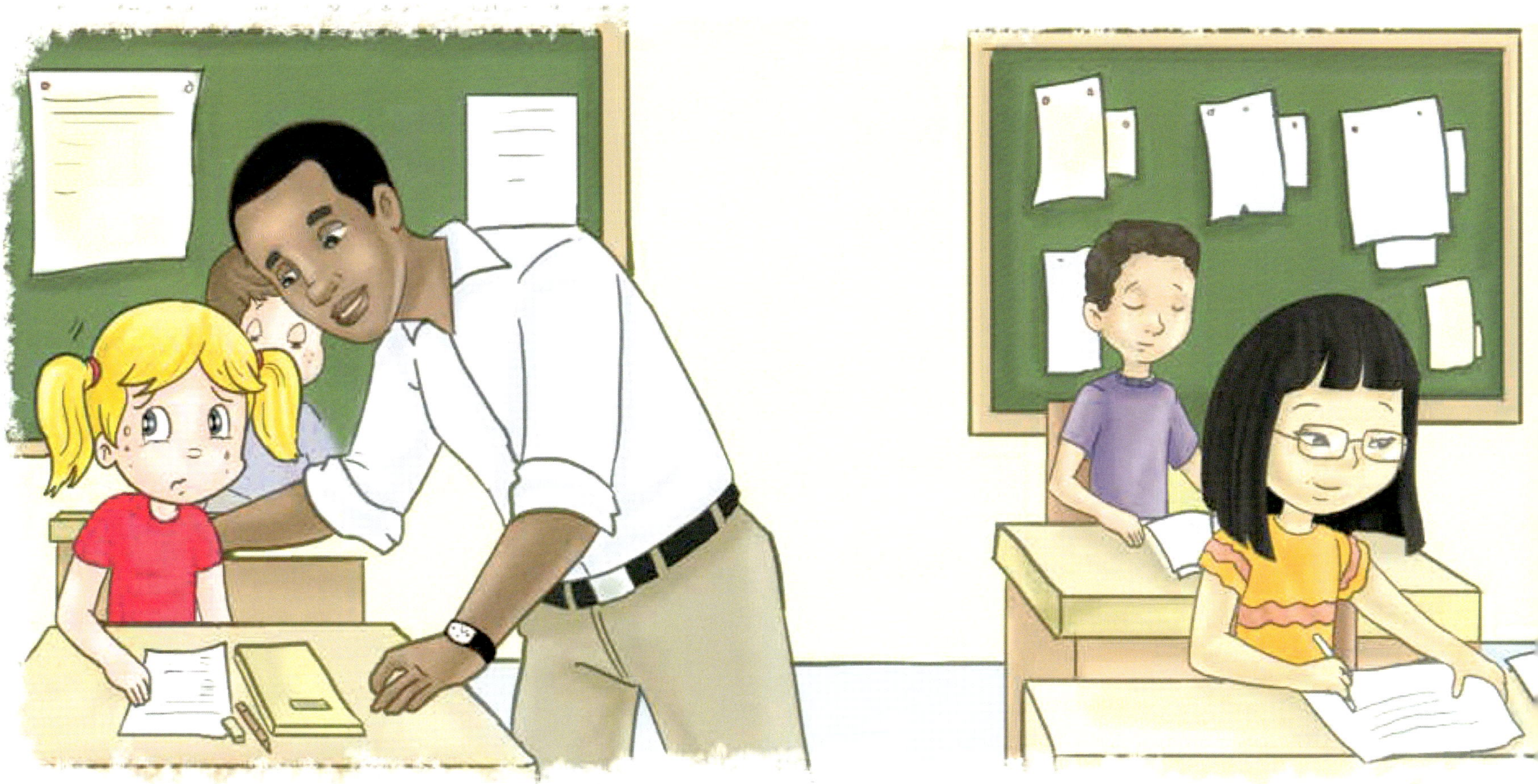

Like many times before, Mr Jones noticed I wasn't focusing on my work. "You seem like you're somewhere else, Susie," said Mr Jones in his usual gentle tone.

But that day, Mr Jones did something he had never done before.

When the test was over, he called for my parents, mom and my step-dad Joe, who I call "dad", to come to school.

I was so worried he was going to complain to mom and dad about my bad grades and they would be mad at me. I really didn't want to be grounded.

After school, Mr Jones, mom and dad had their meeting. While they were talking, I burned some rubber on my sneakers, pacing back and forth, and chewed on my nails.

I felt very anxious.

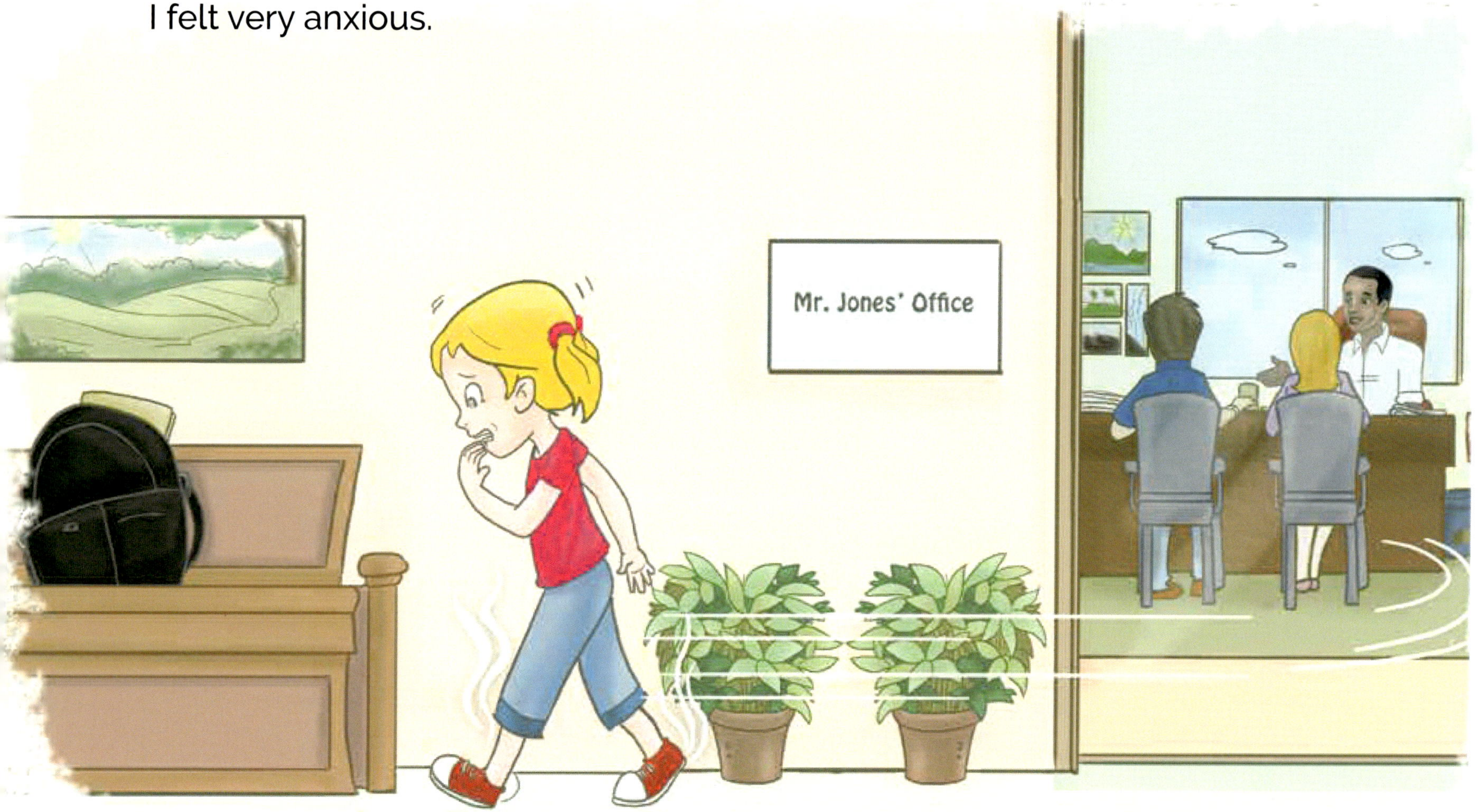

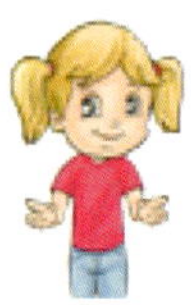

Have you ever felt anxious?
What do you do when you feel anxious?
Do you also pace back and forth or chew on your nails like I do?

When they *finally* came out, Mom put her arm around me and said, Everything is okay, Susie."

Phew! What a relief!

But what did they talk about then? Hmmm...

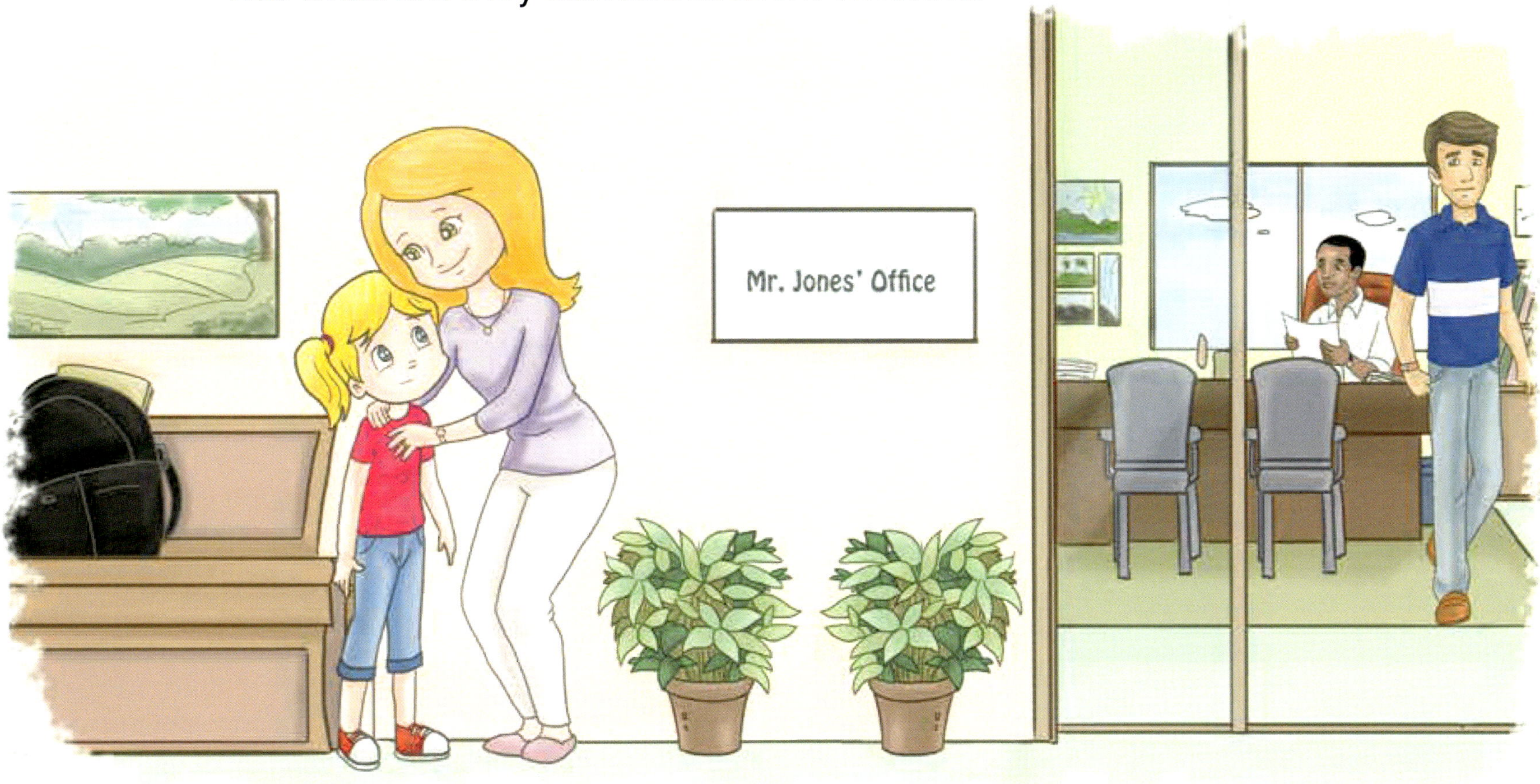

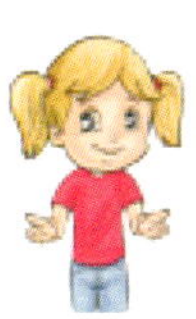

Have you ever felt confused, anxious or suspicious all at the same time? When you experience more than one feeling at the same time, it's called **mixed** feelings.

On the way home, mom and dad told me what the discussion was about.

Mr Jones told them he was concerned about me. He said he had tutored me in science for several months and yet my grades had not improved. He believed I could do really well in science and school in general, but for some reason I was not.

"Also, the other kids often don't include Susie in group projects and she doesn't put forth the effort to make friends either," Mr Jones said.

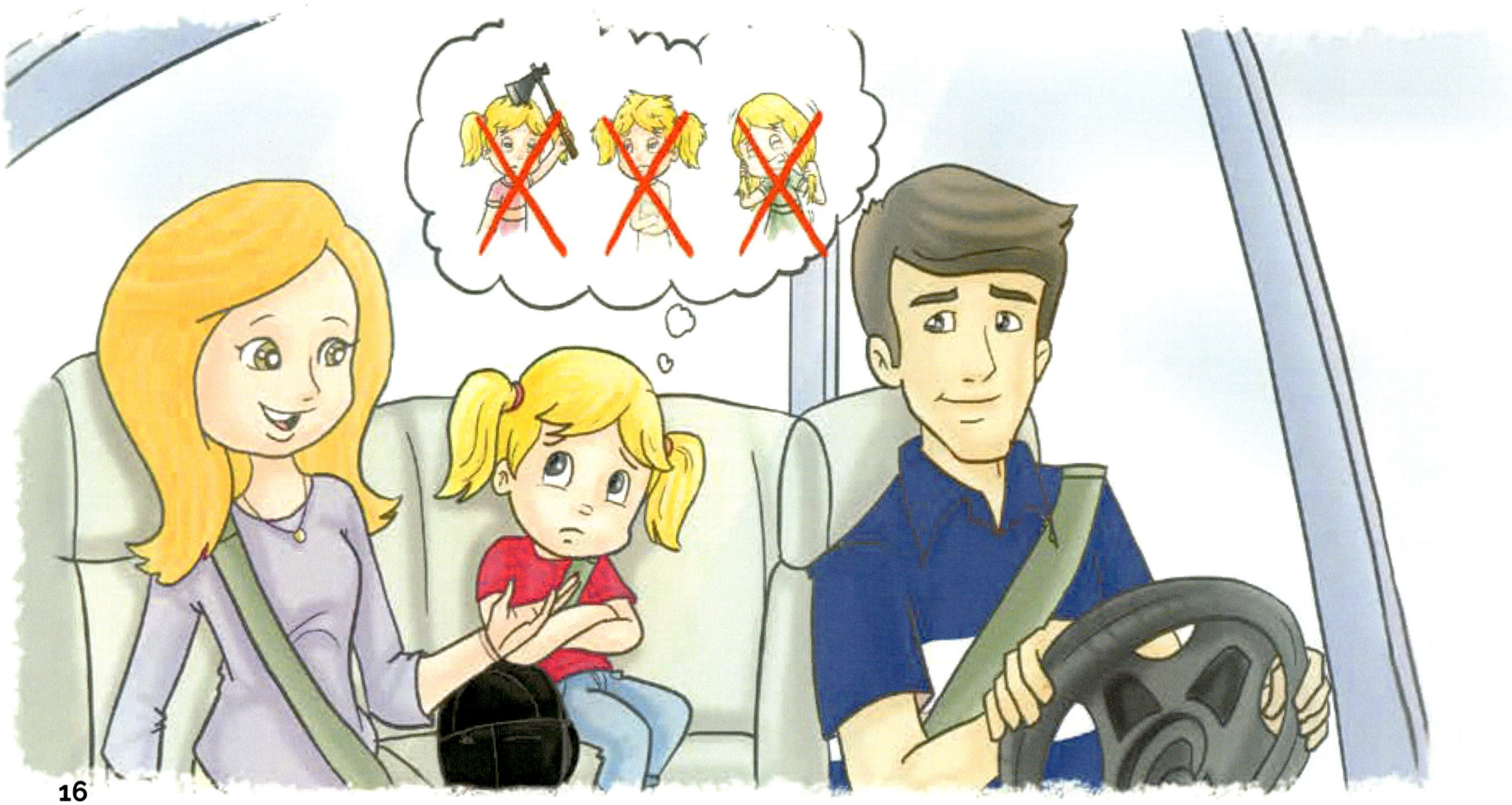

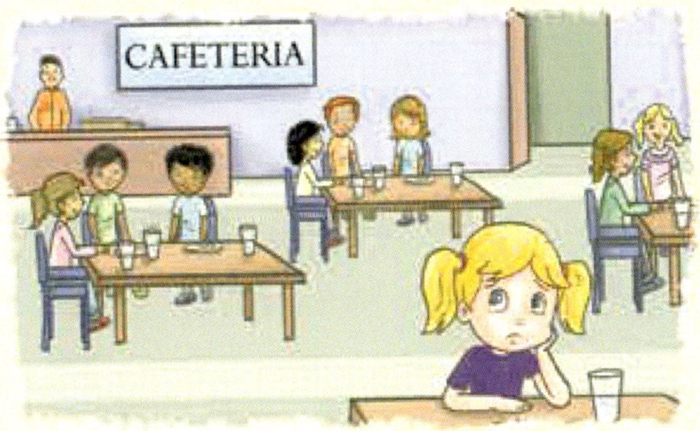

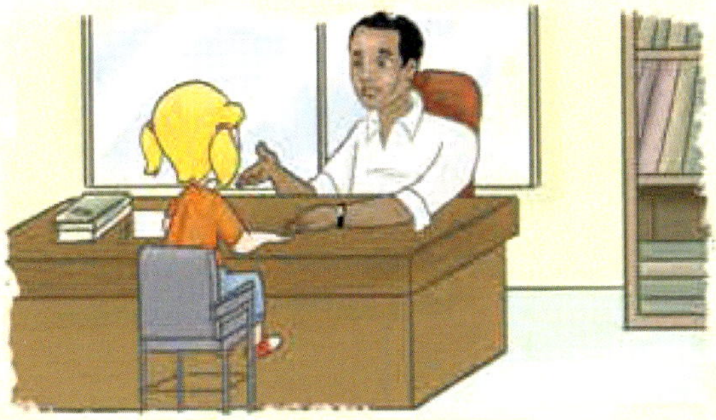

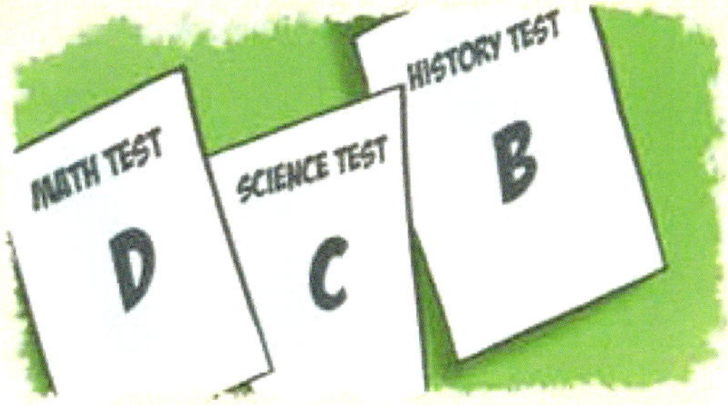

He went on to say, "A lot of the time, she looks spaced out in class. I'm not sure what is going on."

"However, I do know that counselors are really good at helping kids and families in these types of situations. I think it would be a really good idea for Susie and you to go see one."

Grrrr. . . Can you believe that???

I was so upset with Mr Jones! Only crazy people see counselors. I'm not **CRAZY!!!** I'm not **NUTS!!!** Why should **I** have to go see a counselor???

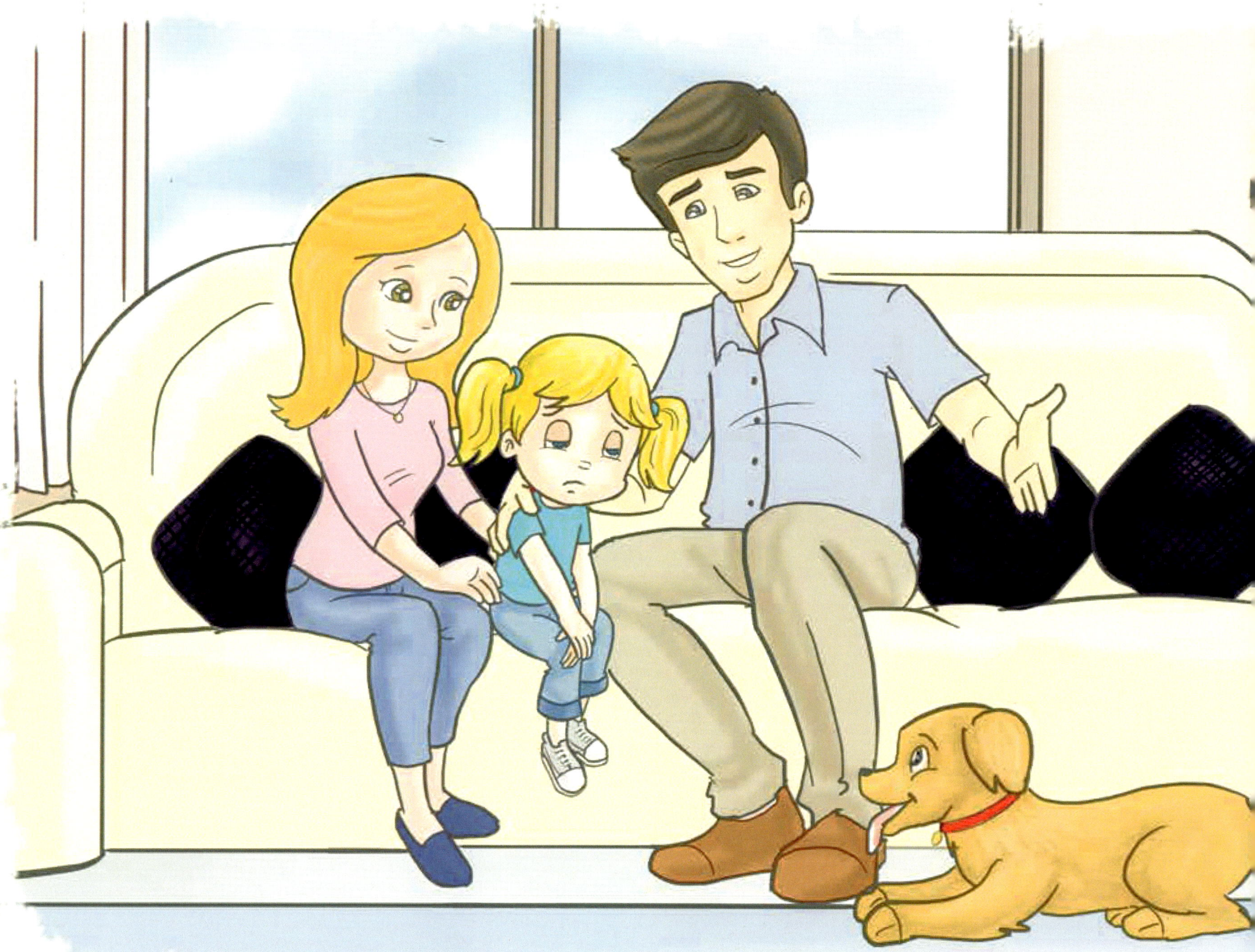

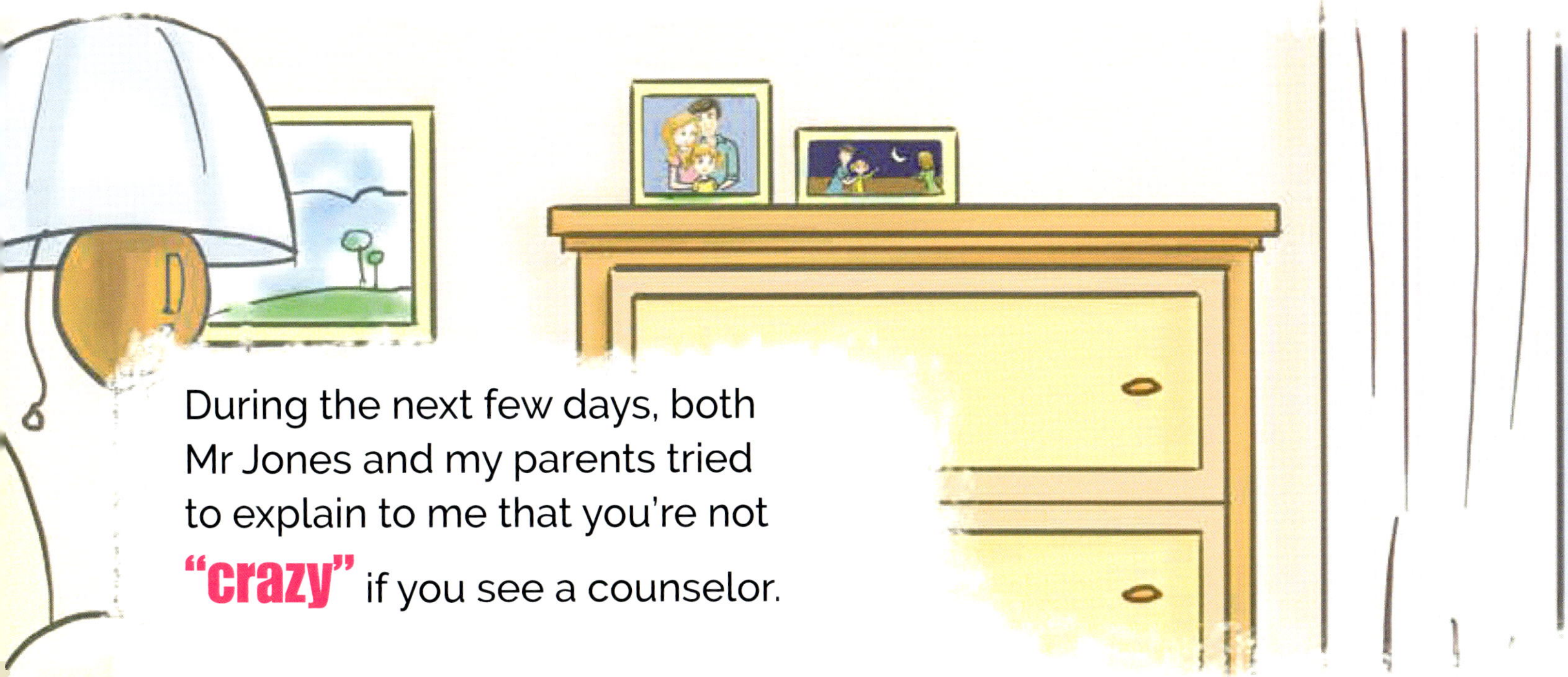

During the next few days, both Mr Jones and my parents tried to explain to me that you're not **"crazy"** if you see a counselor.

"It is absolutely normal and okay to go see one. Everyone can benefit from seeing a counselor," they said.

"We don't quite understand why you space out during class, Susie, and we are worried that you are not making friends. We aren't sure if you are suffering, but our guess is that it probably doesn't feel so good to be in your situation.

We'd like to help but we don't know how.

We have heard of a counselor who has helped many parents like us help their kids feel better. It would be nice for all of us to go together as a family.

We hope you will give us a chance to help you. We truly believe you can do better in school. We think you may be happier if things were different from how they are now."

This was true. Secretly, I did wish things would be different, but I did not share this with anyone, certainly not my parents. I was afraid people would find out I was weird.

Despite wanting things to be different, I really didn't want to go see a counselor. So I told Mom I didn't feel like going. Mom would not take "no" for an answer. She said I needed to go at least once to try it and after the first visit I "could choose not to go again".

I was not happy about it but agreed to go to **ONLY** one appointment.

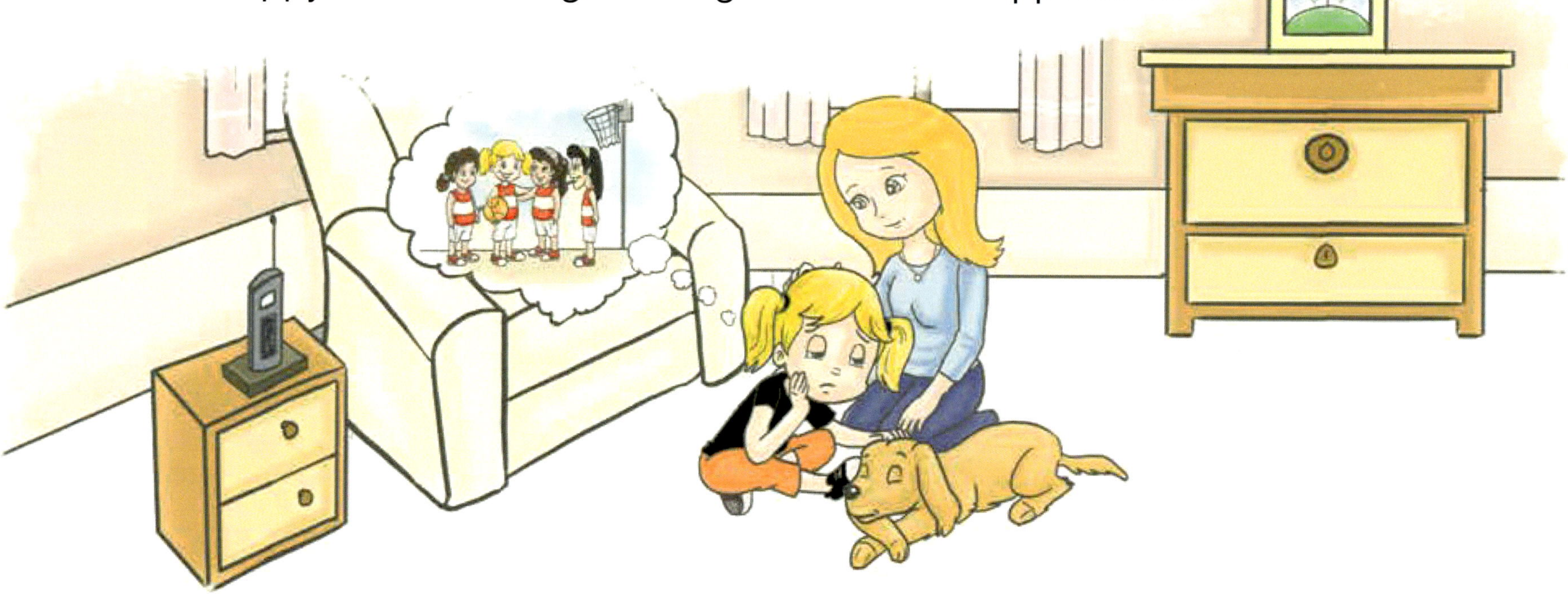

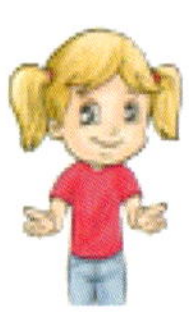

Do you know what it feels like when someone says something is good for you but you still don't want to do it?

I felt scared about meeting this stranger that my parents wanted me to meet.

Will she do anything to me, like give me shots?

What will she ask me to do?

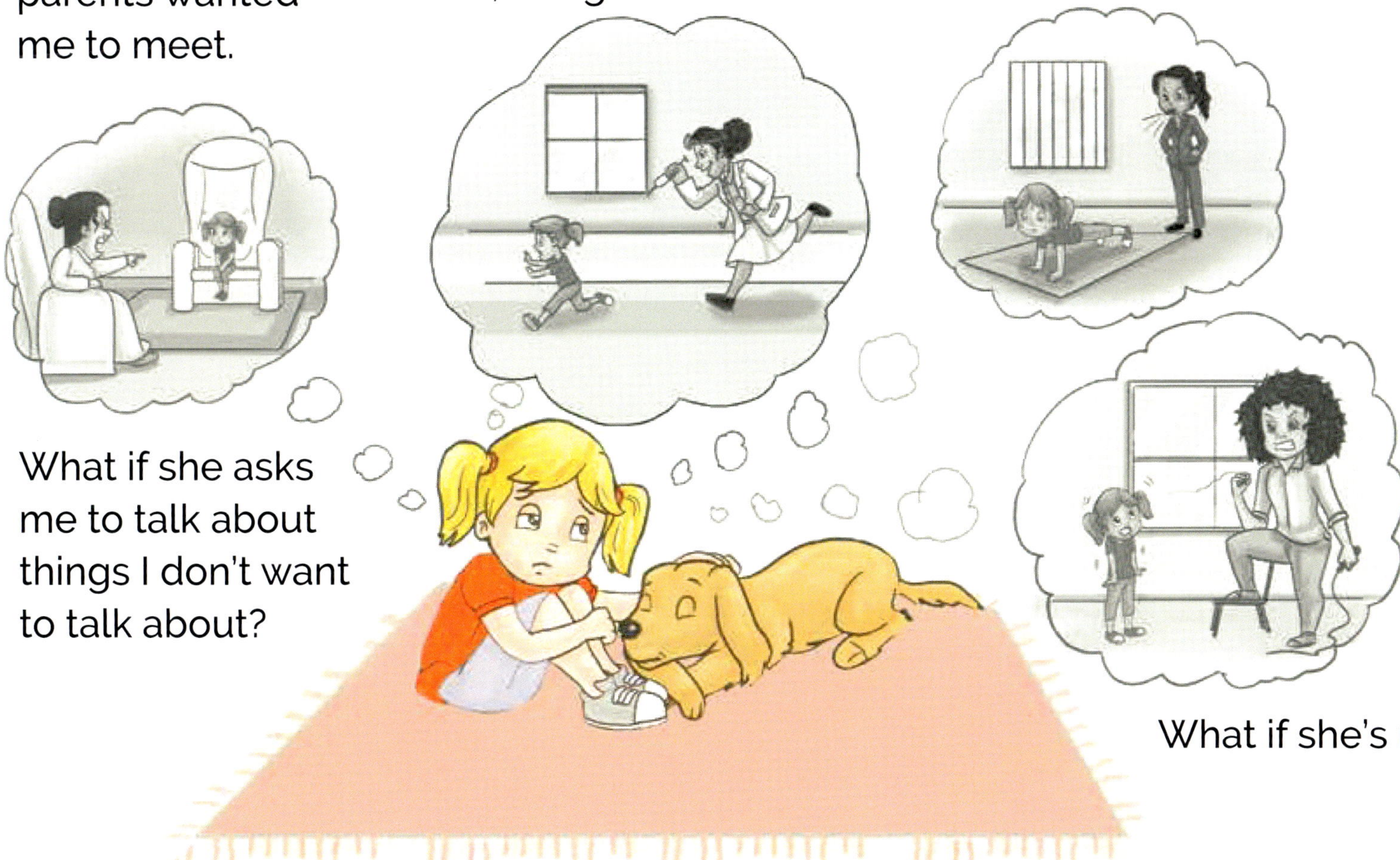

What if she asks me to talk about things I don't want to talk about?

What if she's mean?

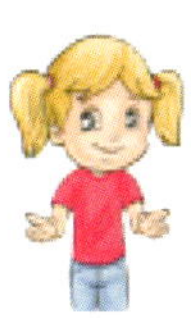

Have you ever had to do something you really didn't want to do?
Did you or would you feel scared seeing a counselor for the first time?
How did you feel the first time you met your counselor?

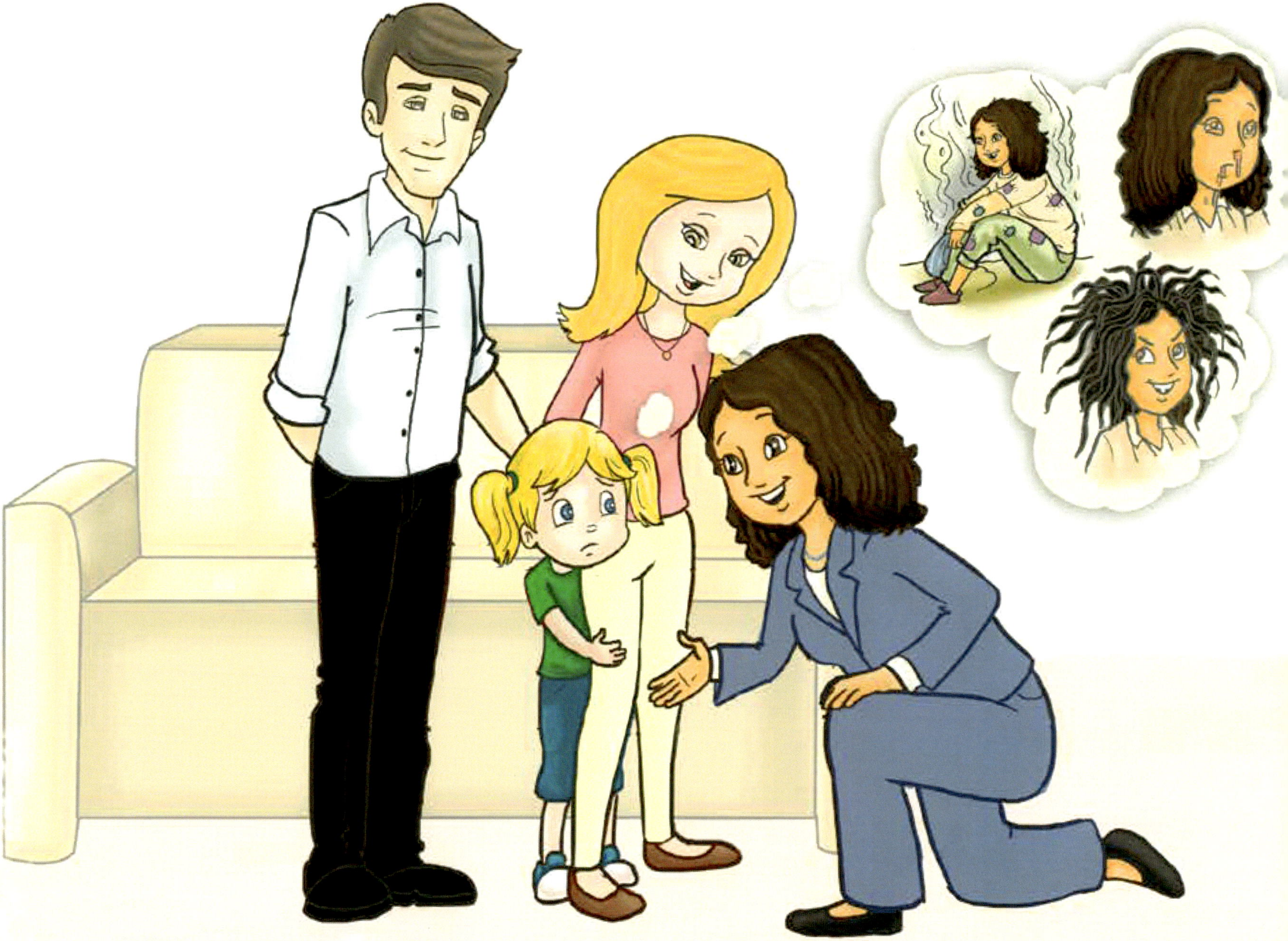

The day for my appointment came.

Mom and dad picked me up after school and we went straight to the counselor's office.

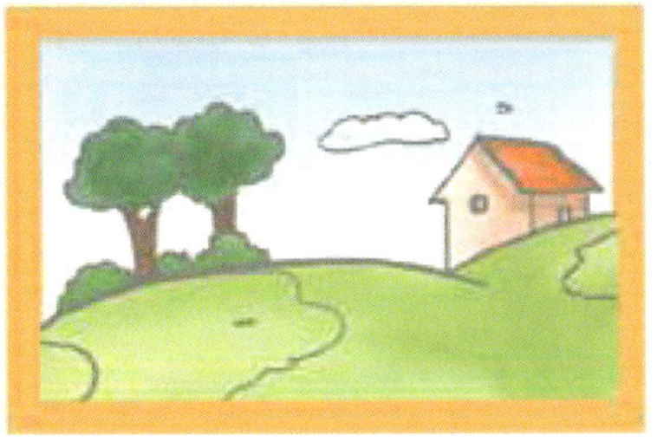

Amy, the counselor, was expecting us. She greeted us with a smile and a friendly "Hello." Mom and dad shook hands with her. Then, Amy leaned over to say a special "Hello" to me.

I was surprised she didn't smell bad.

She didn't have drool or snot on her face and, in fact, she didn't even look STRANGE, **MEAN** or scary!

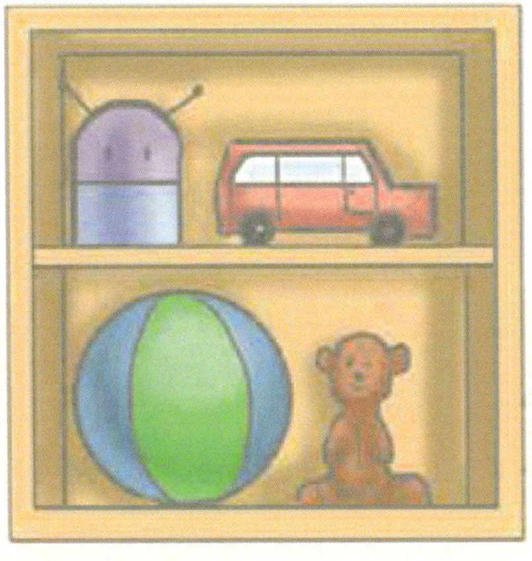

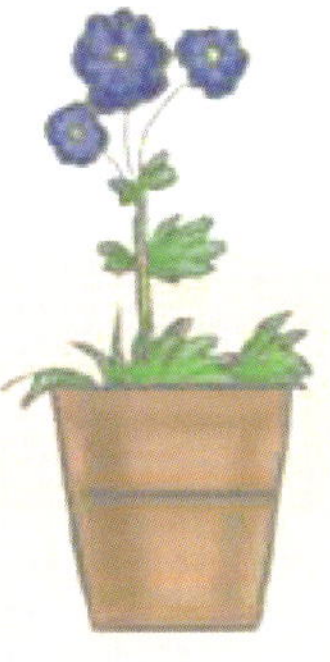

"She *looks* alright but who knows what she's **REALLY** like," I thought to myself.

Although I did not feel like being friendly, I quickly gathered my thoughts and said "Hello" back. I did not want to make my parents unhappy by behaving rudely.

We entered Amy's office.

I did a quick scan of her room. It looked clean and neat and didn't have any of those scary tools and instruments I had seen in my regular doctor's office.

Believe it or not, Amy's office looked like a fun place. It had toys, games and art materials too!

Most importantly, there didn't seem to be any needles lying around.

But I still wasn't completely sure.

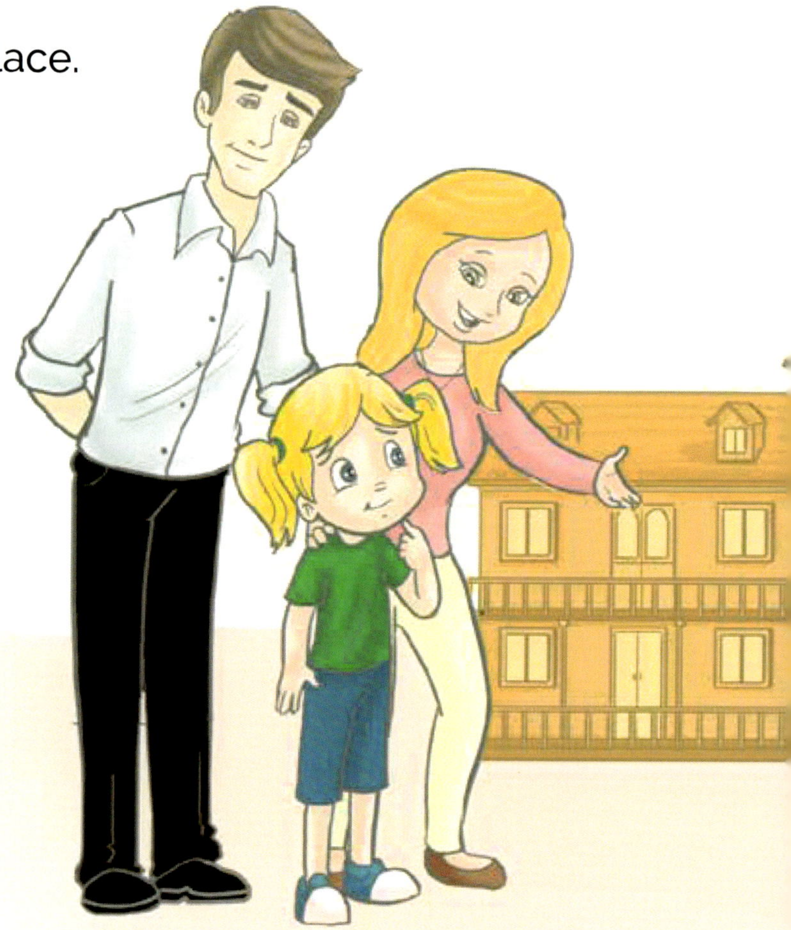

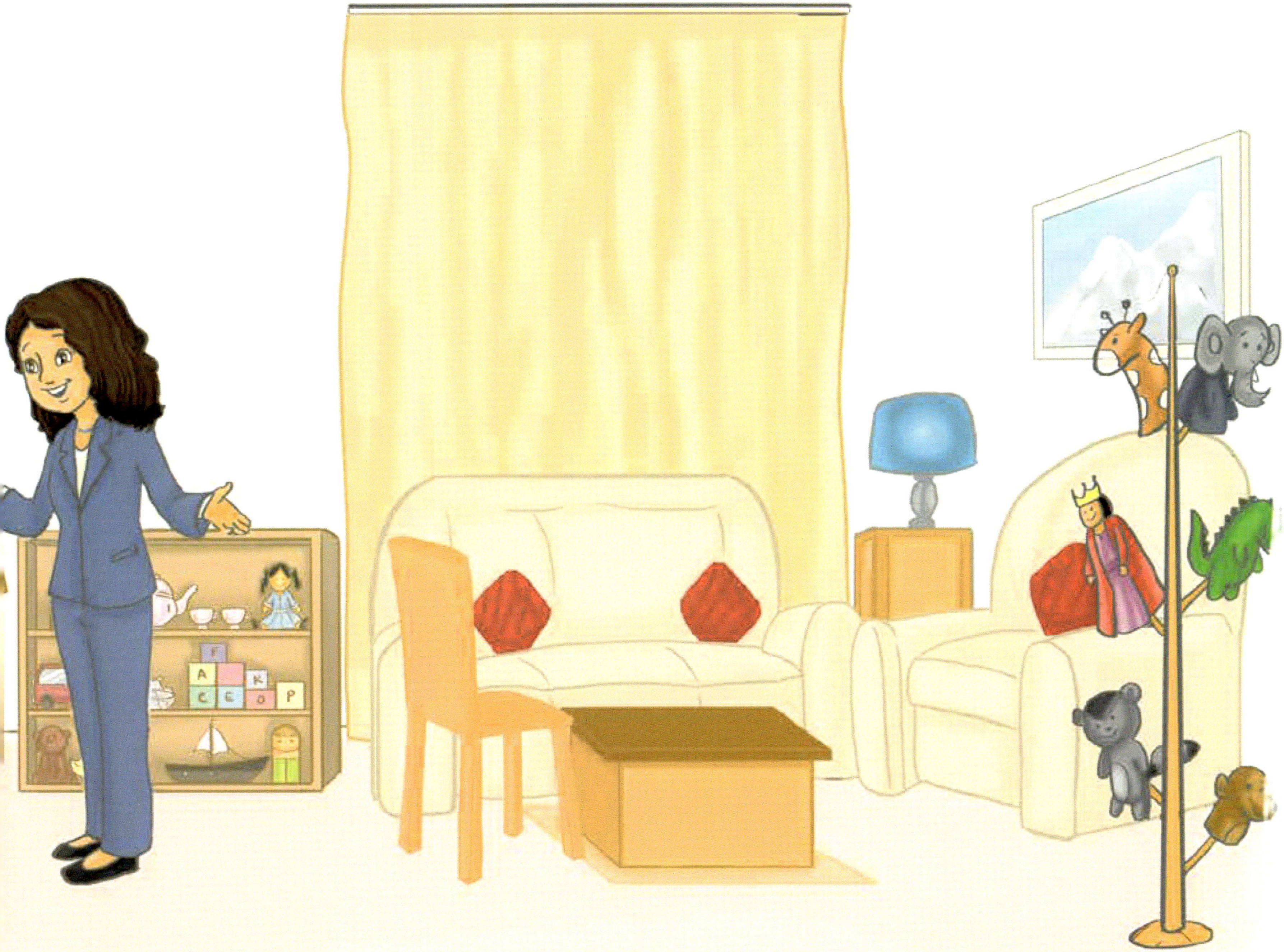

Once we settled into the office, Amy told us, “Things you share with me will be kept private, except in special circumstances. You are welcome to talk about anything under the sun and you can ask me about anything at all too.”

Then Amy turned to me and said, “If you feel like it you can draw, paint, or play with the toys in the room. And if you don't feel like talking at all, that's okay too.”

“This whole counseling thing is starting to sound better than I expected,” I thought.

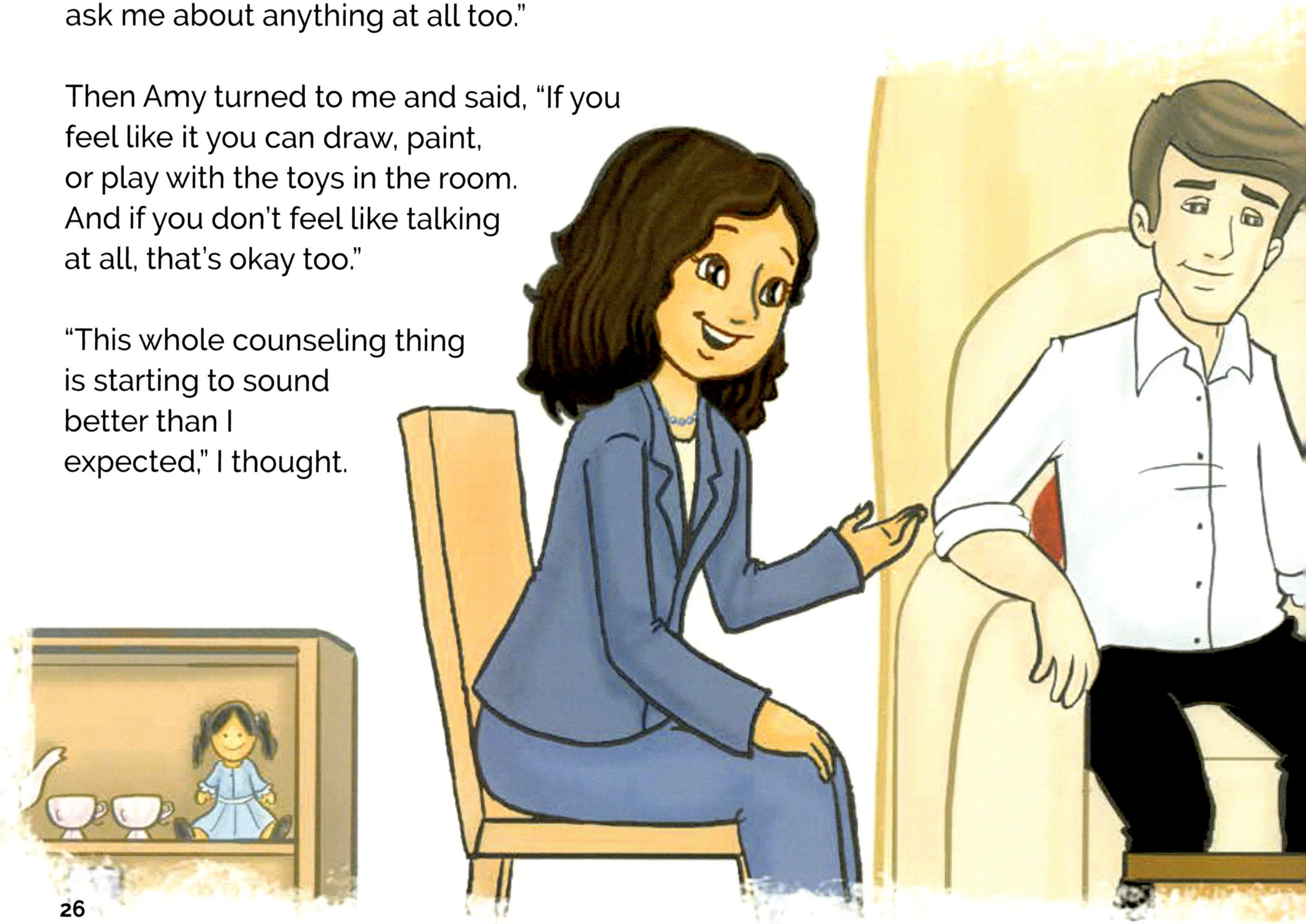

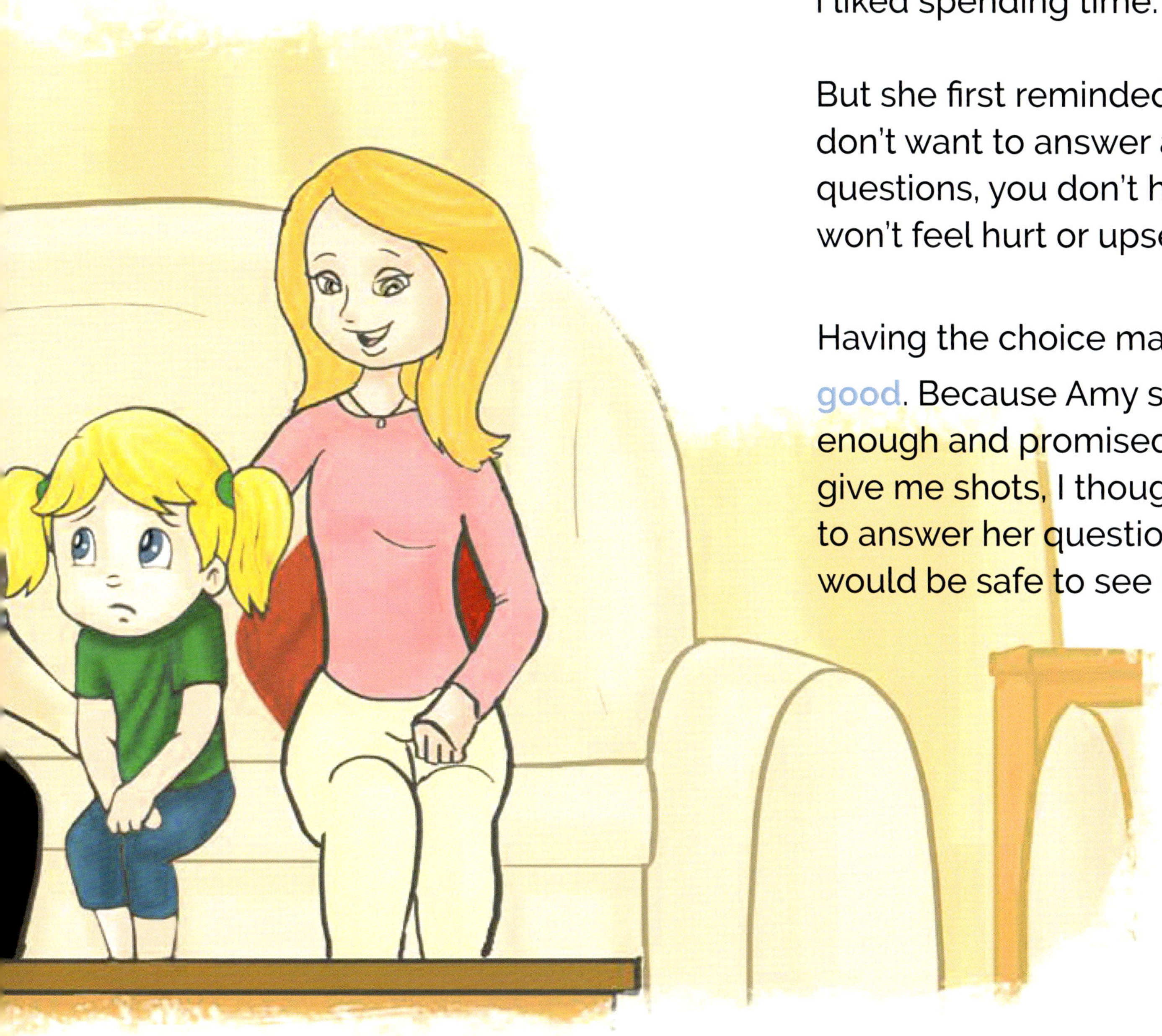

As our meeting went on, Amy asked me about school and friends. She wanted to know what I liked and disliked about school, and with whom I liked spending time.

But she first reminded me, "If you don't want to answer any of my questions, you don't have to. And I won't feel hurt or upset."

Having the choice made me feel good. Because Amy seemed nice enough and promised she would not give me shots, I thought it was okay to answer her questions and that it would be safe to see her again.

I ended up seeing Amy the next week and the week after that too.

I wasn't totally sure about her for a while, but as time went on, I realized she wasn't as bad as I had expected.

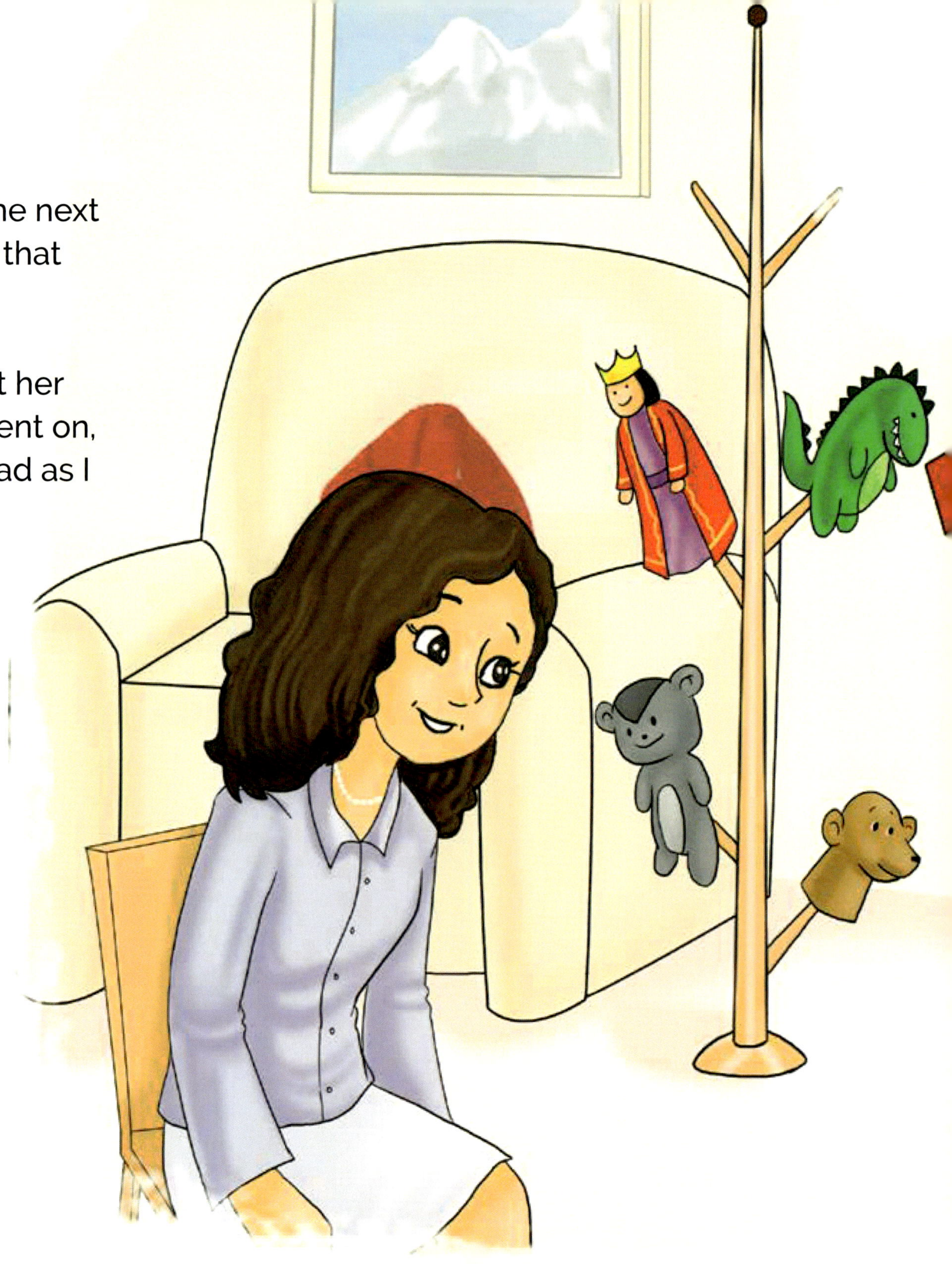

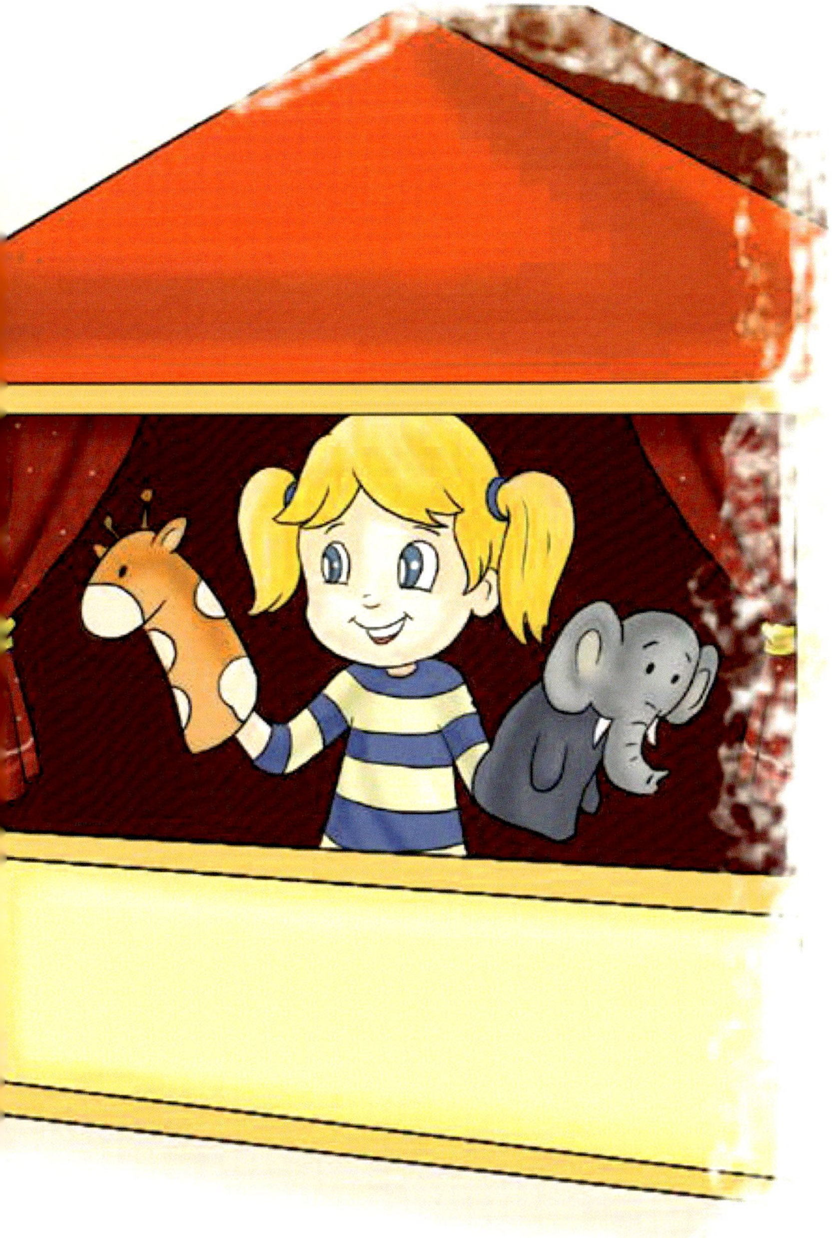

And, to my surprise, I began to notice I was actually starting to like Amy.

I decided to meet with her every week.

Amy was very kind and did not think badly about anything I did or said. Even after my parents told her, “Susie keeps to herself and her mind tends to wander,” Amy didn’t think badly of me!

But still, I was afraid to tell her about something that was bothering me. I was afraid she’d find out I was

WEIRD.

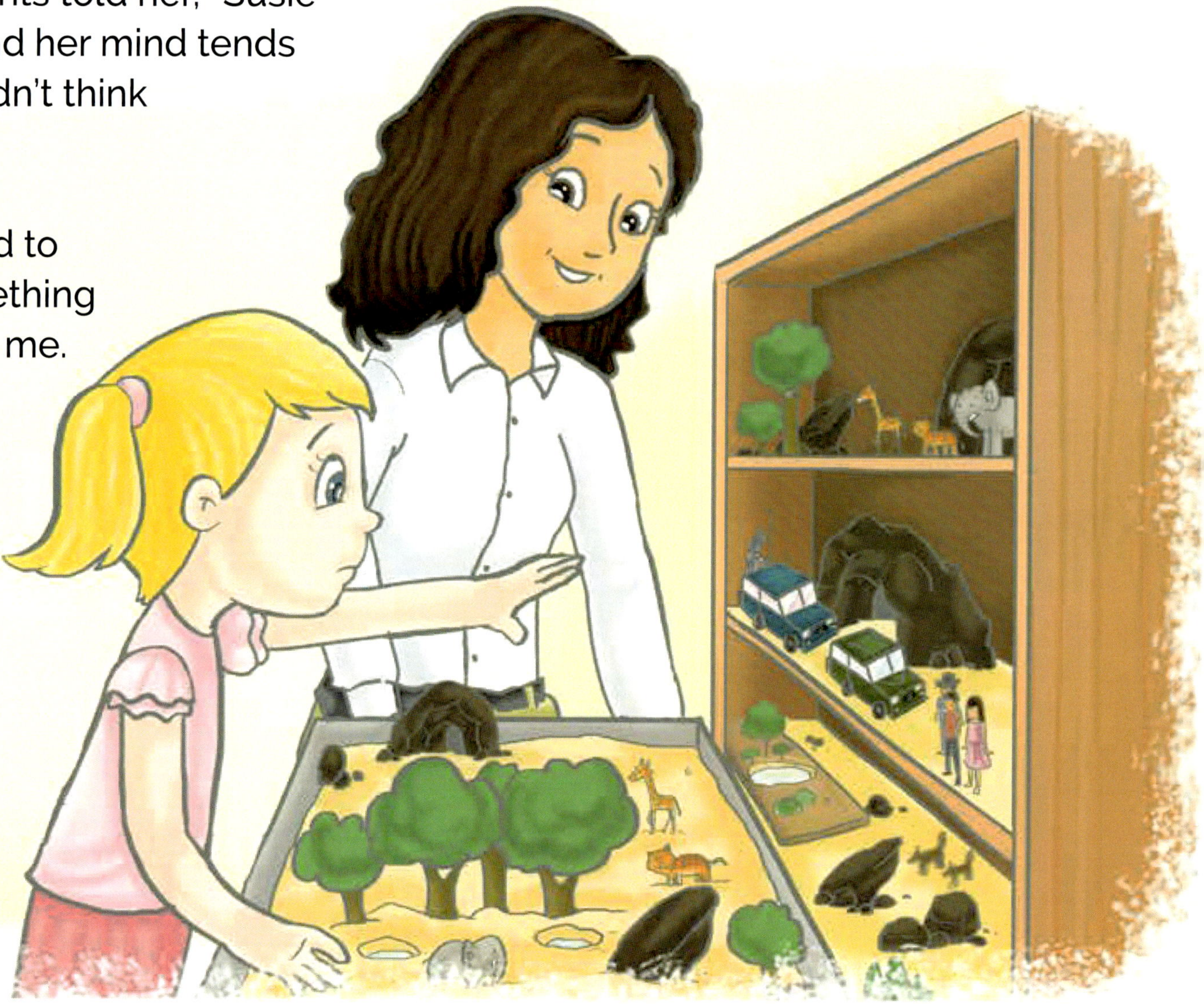

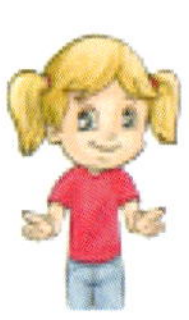

Can you guess what it was that I had such a hard time telling Amy? I hope you won’t think I’m weird. It’s something I have **NEVER, EVER** told anyone.

It was the voice.

I was scared to tell Amy that I heard a voice. It was so hard to talk about.

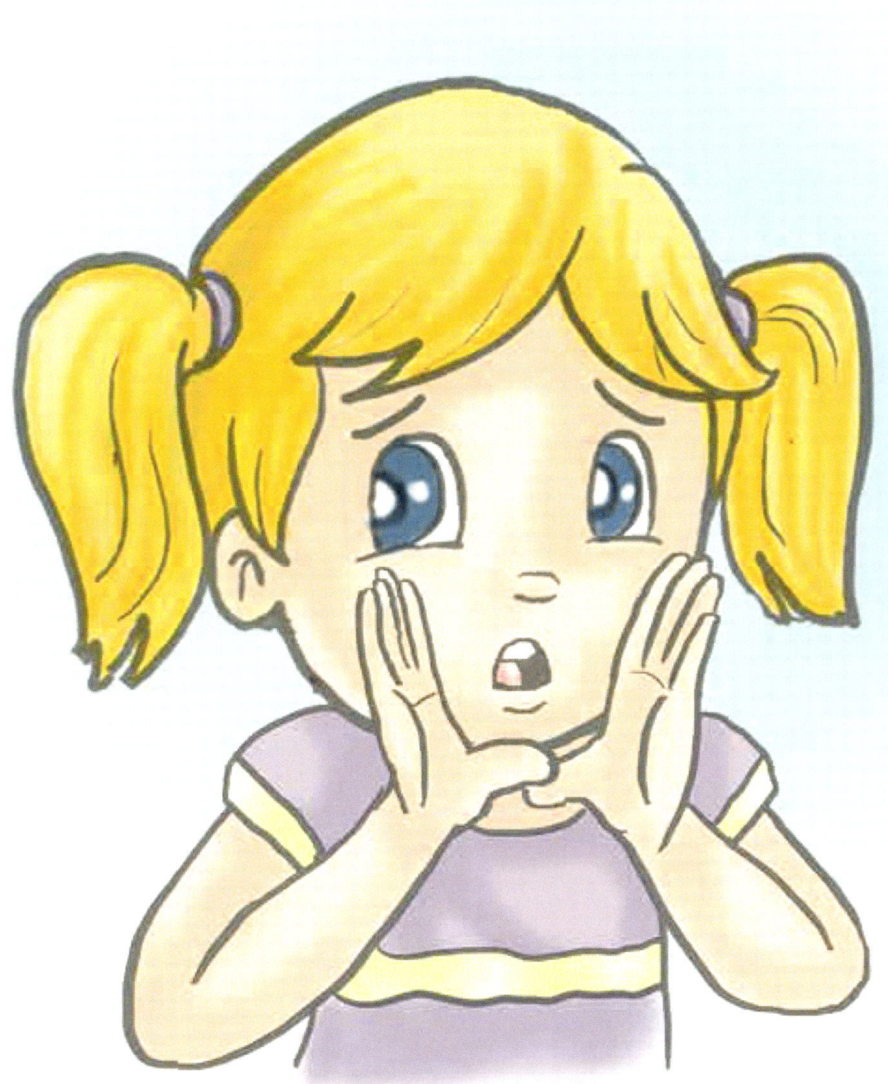

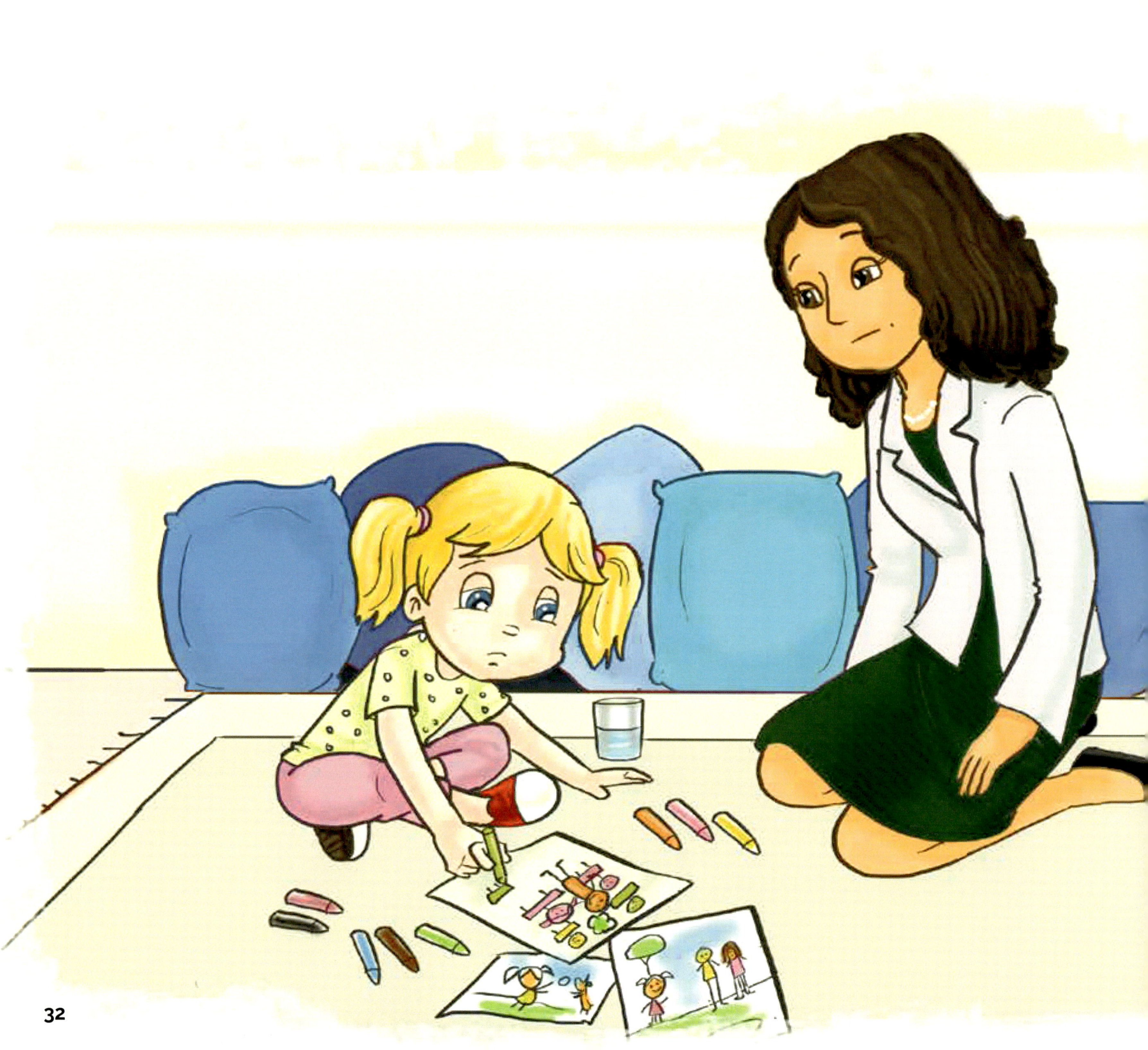

One time, I actually tried to tell Amy about the voice.

I shared with her how my teacher would frequently say, "Smile, Susie! Life's not that bad!" and that, even when I tried my hardest, I couldn't smile. But that was as much as I could say.

I was afraid to go on to tell Amy about the voice that made me feel too sad to smile.

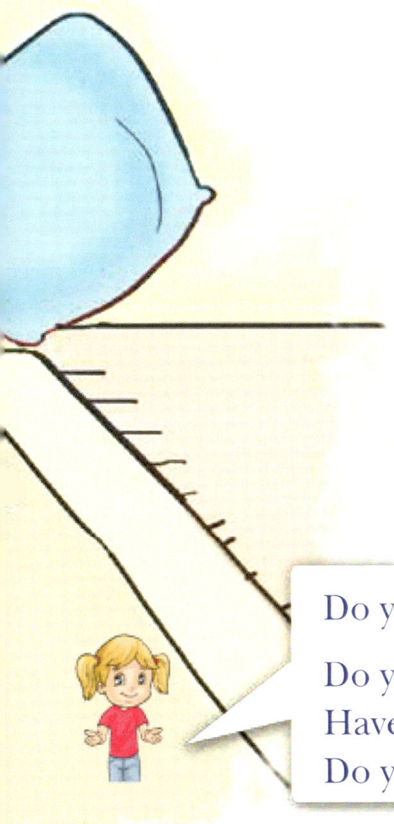

Do you think I am WEIRD?
Do you think I am CRAZY?
Have you ever had a hard time telling a grown-up something?
Do you hear a voice(s) like I do?

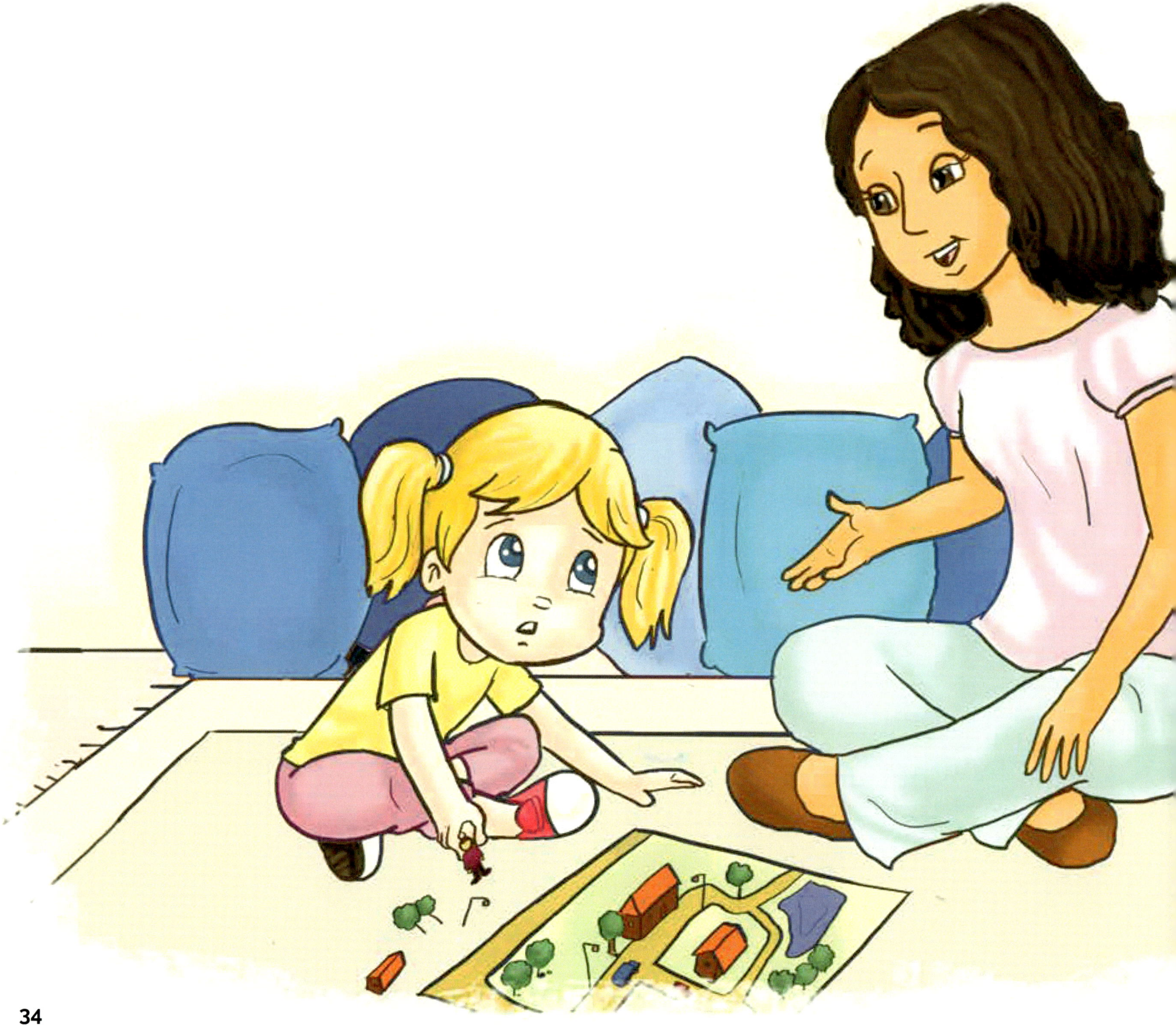

One day, I got so sick of the voice. I made up my mind that somehow I had to do something about it.

So, during one of my meetings with Amy, I gritted my teeth, took several deep breaths and mustered up the courage to talk about it.

I told Amy about the voice.

Amy's reaction surprised me.

She didn't laugh. She didn't appear surprised. She didn't give me the "You're out of your mind" look.

Instead, she said "Tell me more about the voice."

So I told her what I knew and she helped me with the rest.

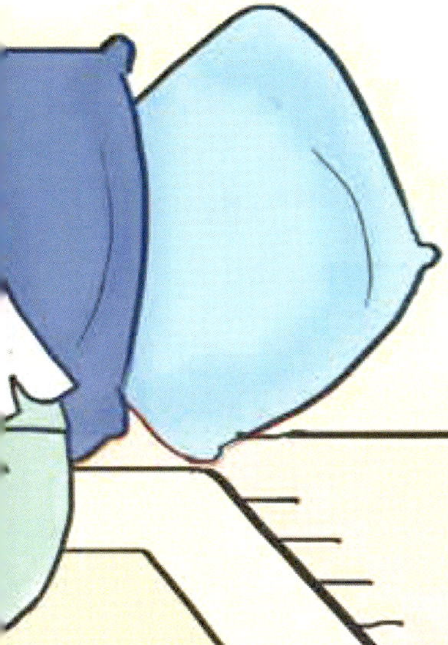

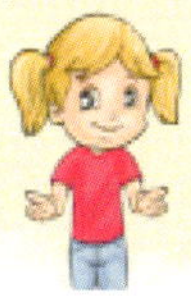

Have you ever tried to gather up all your courage to do something really **BIG**, **SCARY** and **HARD**?
What was it?

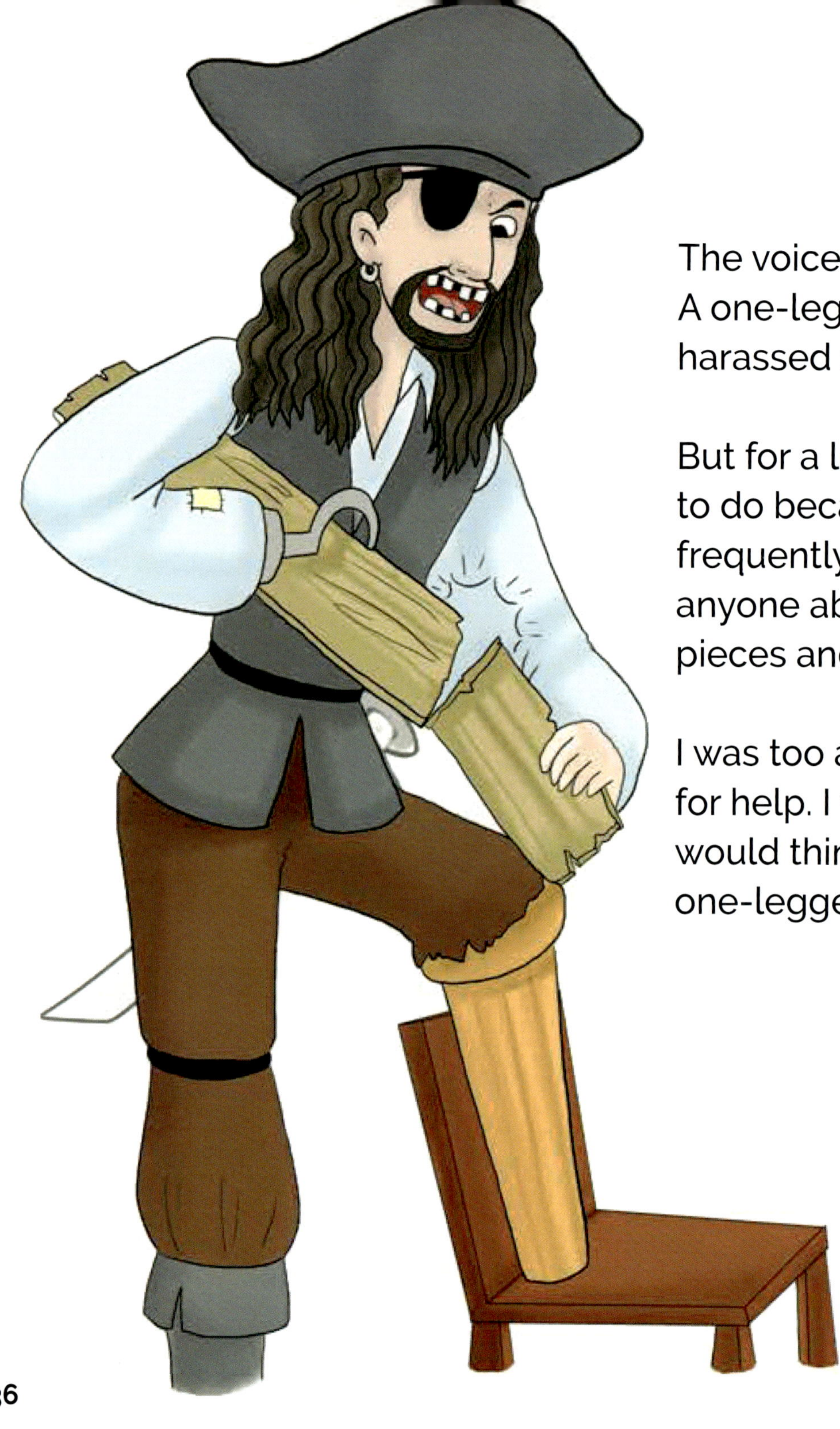

The voice I heard belonged to a man. A one-legged pirate, actually. He harassed me and I wanted him to stop.

But for a long time I didn't know what to do because the one-legged pirate frequently growled, "If you dare tell anyone about me, I'll break you into pieces and you'll look like me!"

I was too afraid to tell anyone or ask for help. I was also worried that people would think it was my fault that the one-legged pirate tormented me.

My voice was a secret for two years before I told Amy.

Amy understood how uncomfortable and helpless the one-legged pirate made me feel.

“If you’d like, we can explore it together to figure out what the one-legged pirate is all about. Then we can see if there is a way you can manage the voice so that you can be happier,” Amy said.

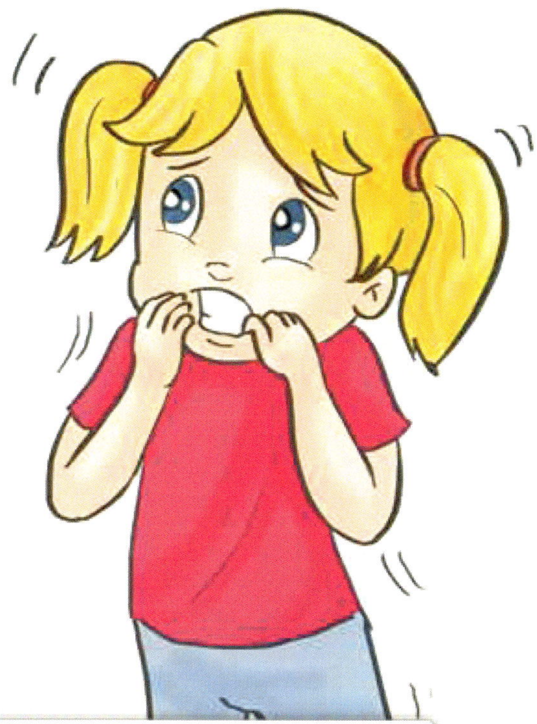

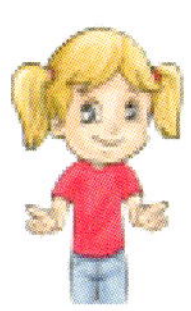

If you hear a voice(s), what is it like?

In order to help me, Amy needed to know more about the voice. She asked me lots of questions so that she could understand what I was hearing and seeing.

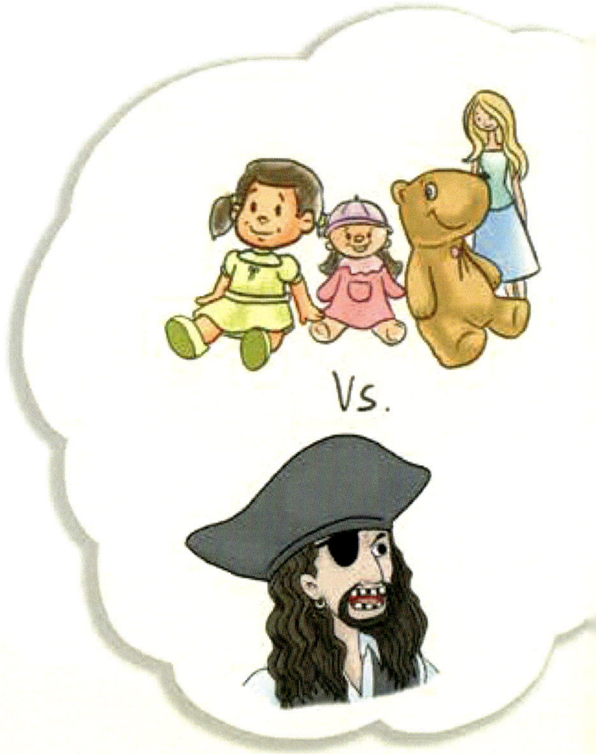

"Does the voice have a shape and figure, or is it just a voice?"

"Is the voice real?"

"How is the voice different from your dolls at home and kids at your school?"

"Is the voice the same or different from when you have a debate with yourself in your head? For example, the debate you have when you're deciding whether to wear a blue or yellow shirt or have macaroni or pizza for dinner."

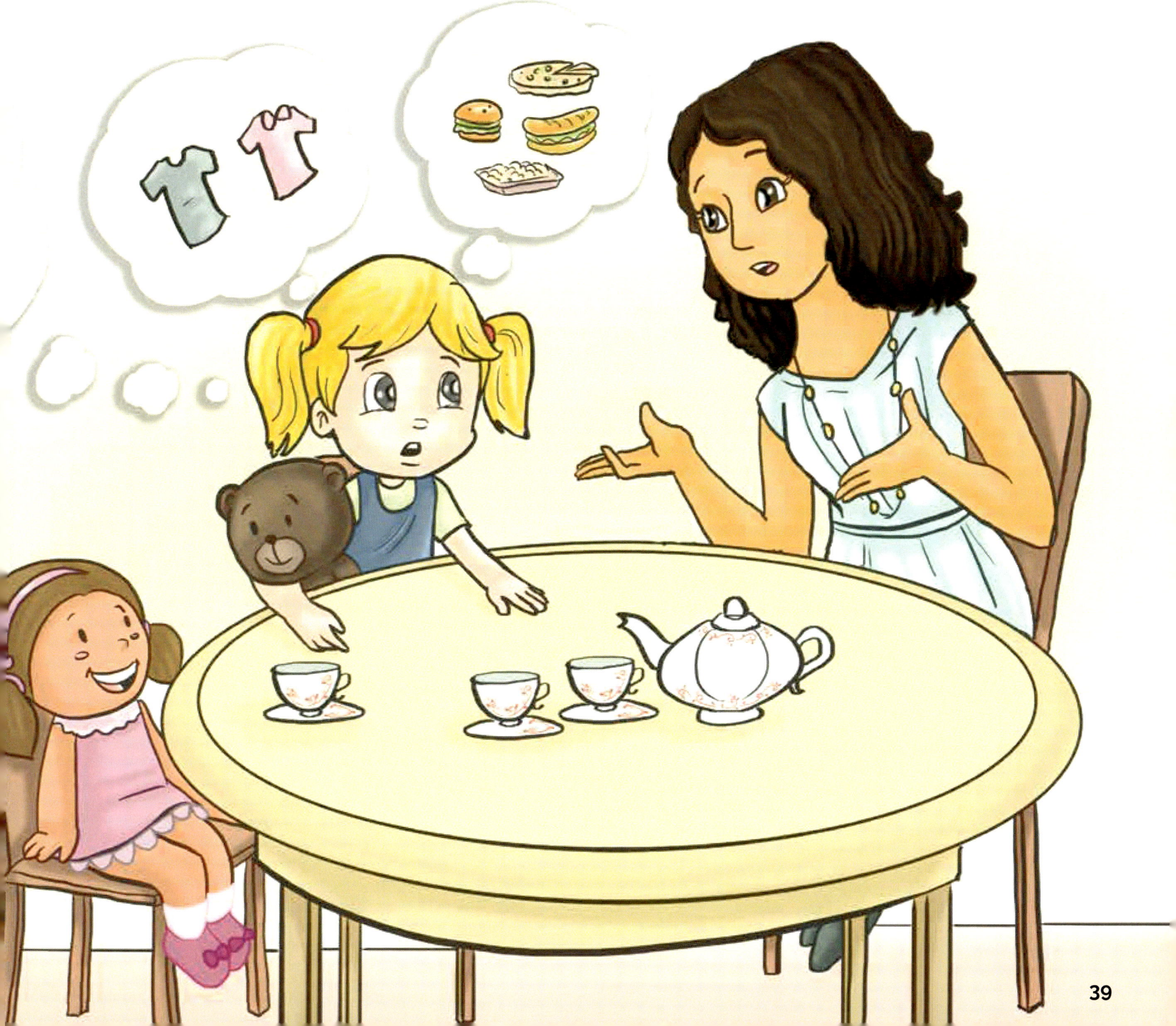

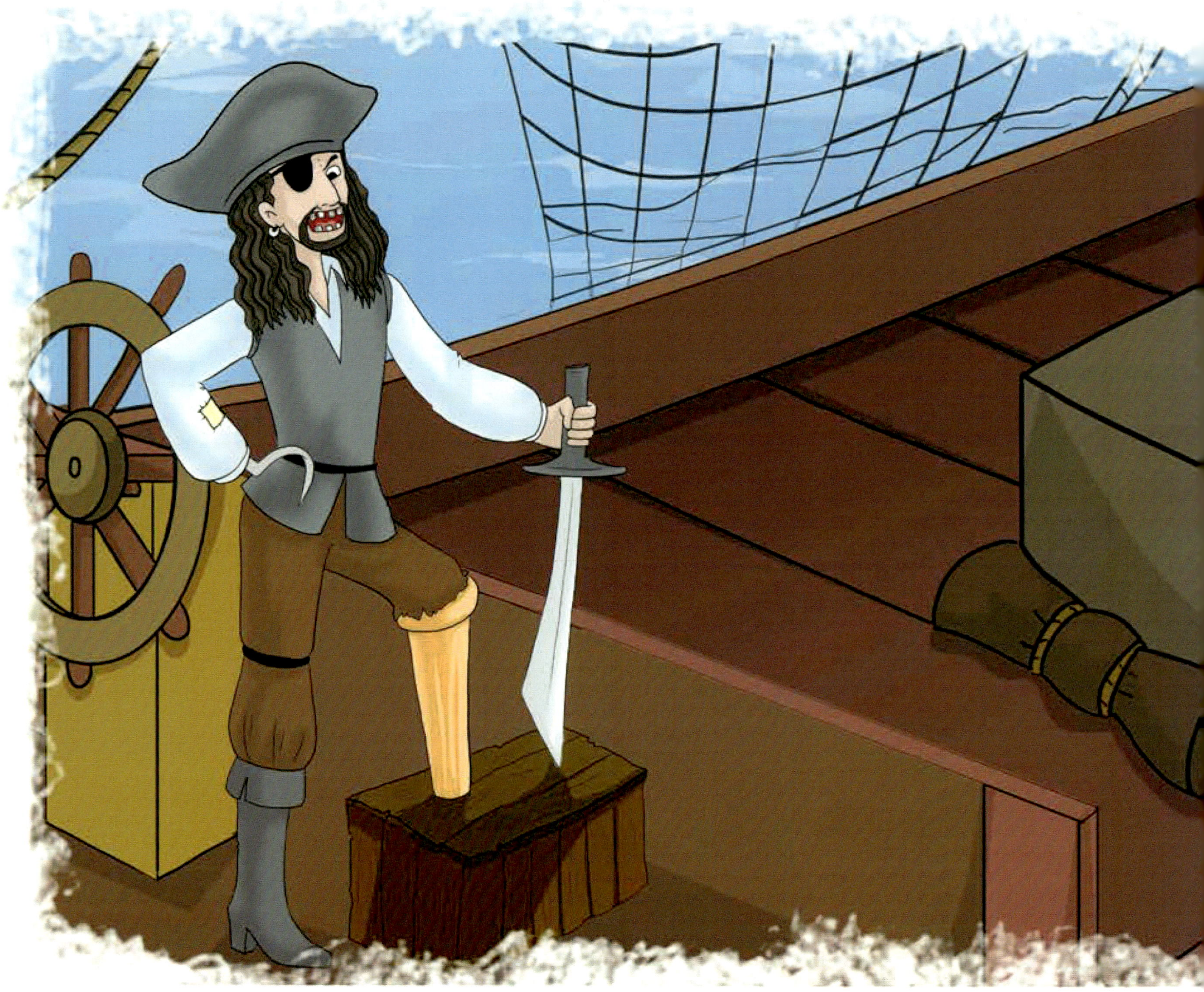

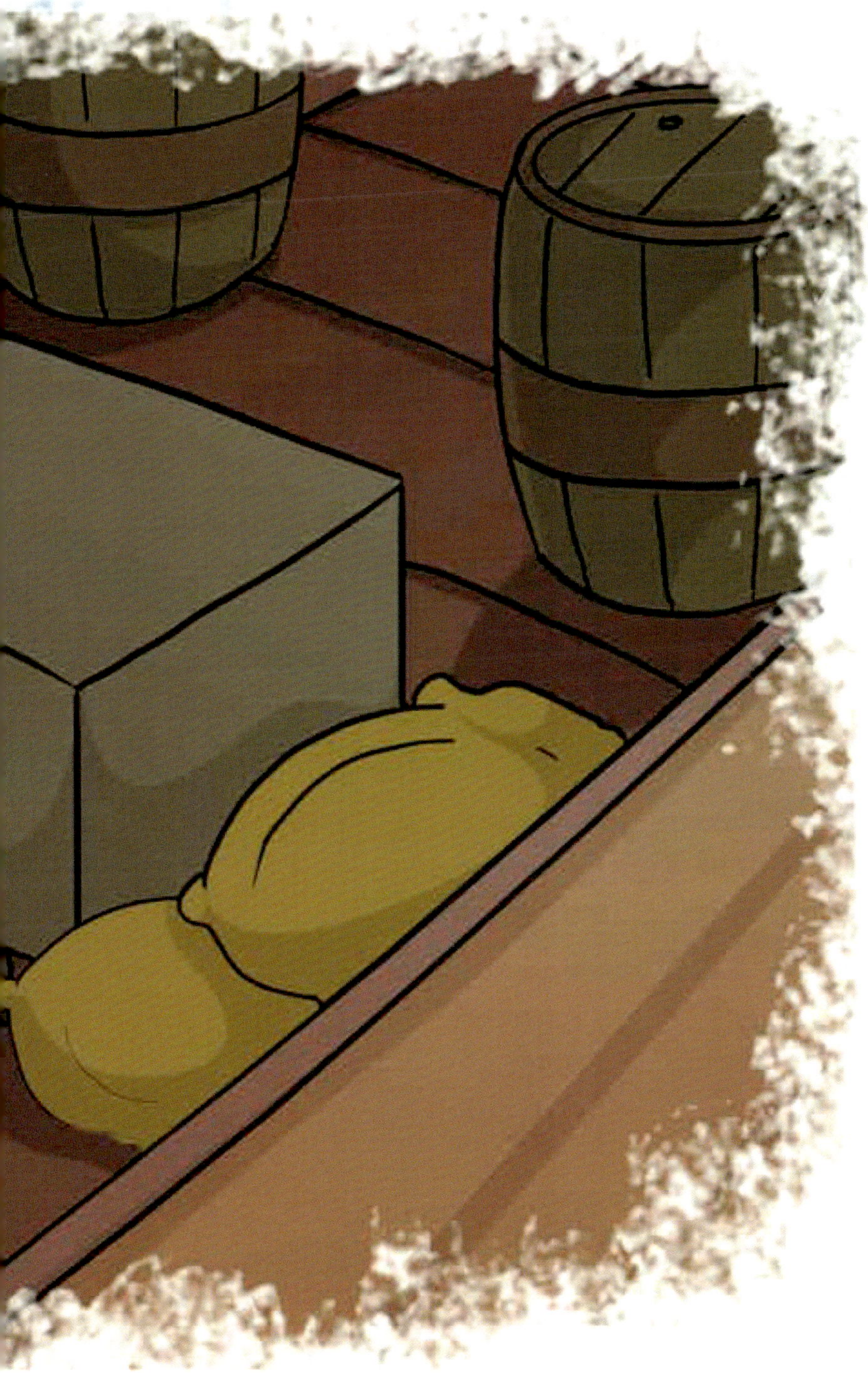

I answered Amy's questions as best as I could.

I told her that I definitely heard the voice and saw what was making it too.

He was a one-legged pirate with a left peg-leg and a hook for his right arm.

He always had on a torn blue shirt and a pair of raggedy pants with one pant leg cropped off.

He had a short beard, wore an earring in just one ear, a patch over his right eye, and had ugly-looking teeth.

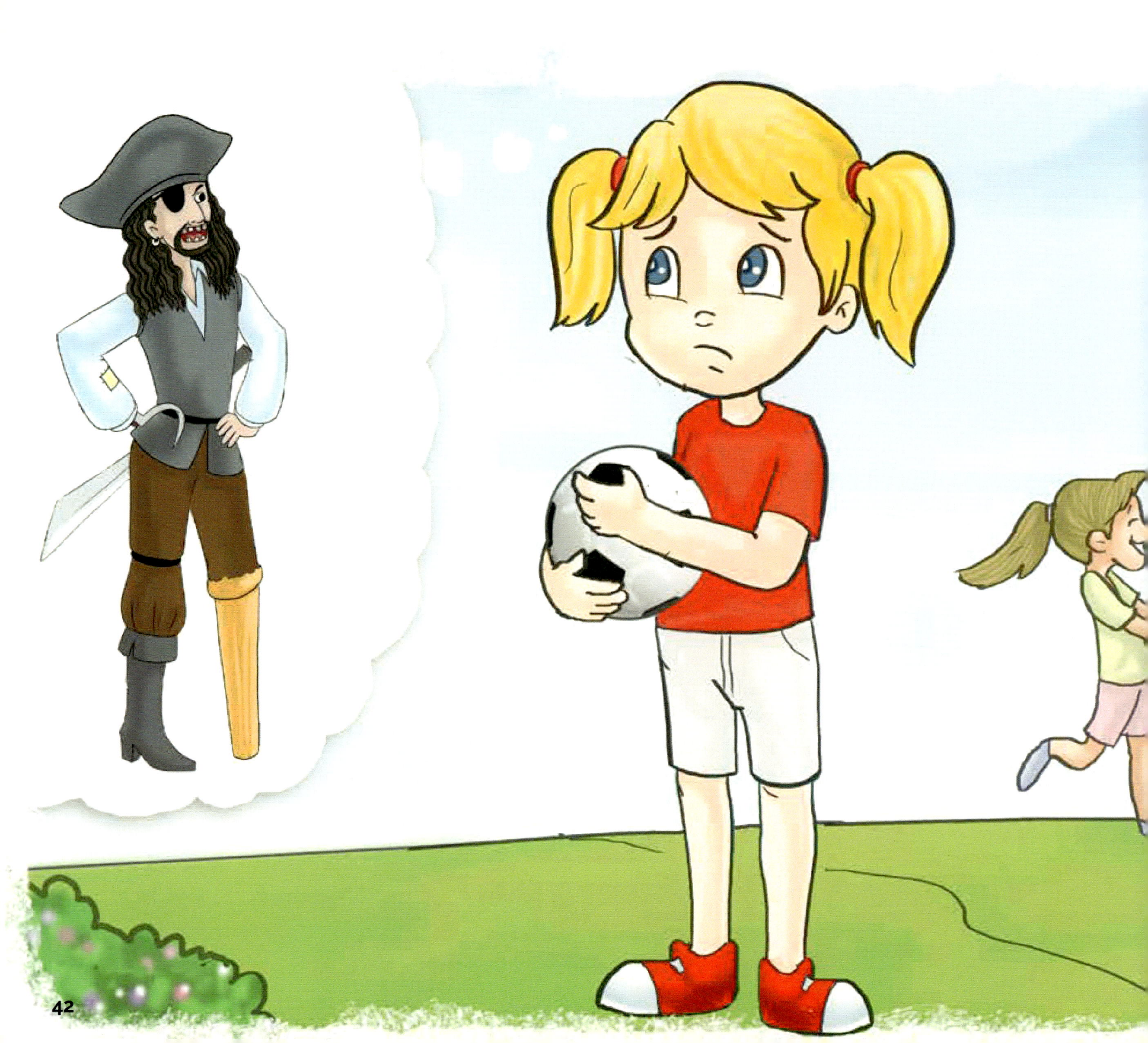

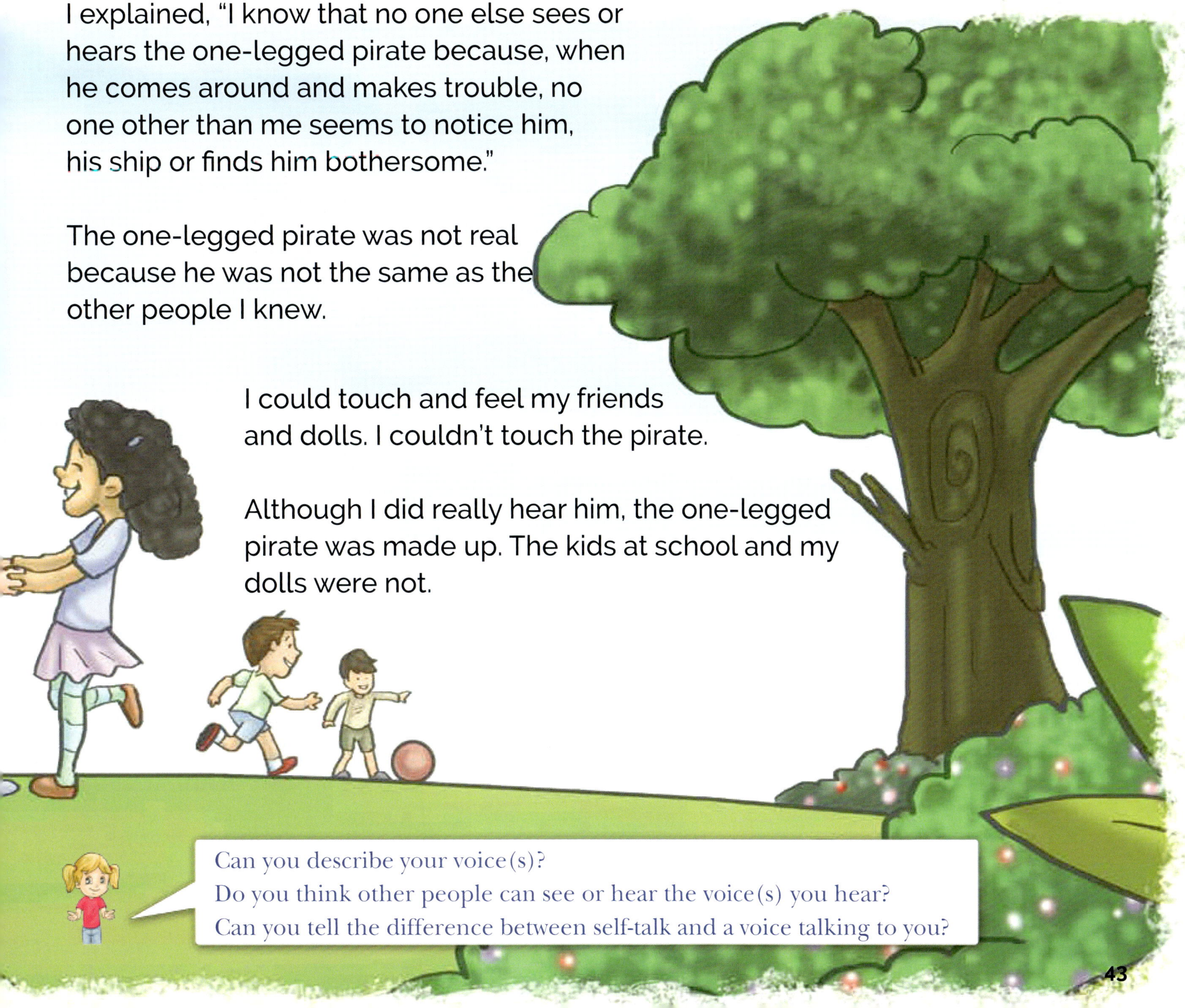

I explained, "I know that no one else sees or hears the one-legged pirate because, when he comes around and makes trouble, no one other than me seems to notice him, his ship or finds him bothersome."

The one-legged pirate was not real because he was not the same as the other people I knew.

I could touch and feel my friends and dolls. I couldn't touch the pirate.

Although I did really hear him, the one-legged pirate was made up. The kids at school and my dolls were not.

Can you describe your voice(s)?
Do you think other people can see or hear the voice(s) you hear?
Can you tell the difference between self-talk and a voice talking to you?

It was hard work talking about the voice.

And just when I thought I was done,
Amy had more questions for me.

"When is the one-legged pirate
the most and least bothersome?"

"How frequently does
he come around?"

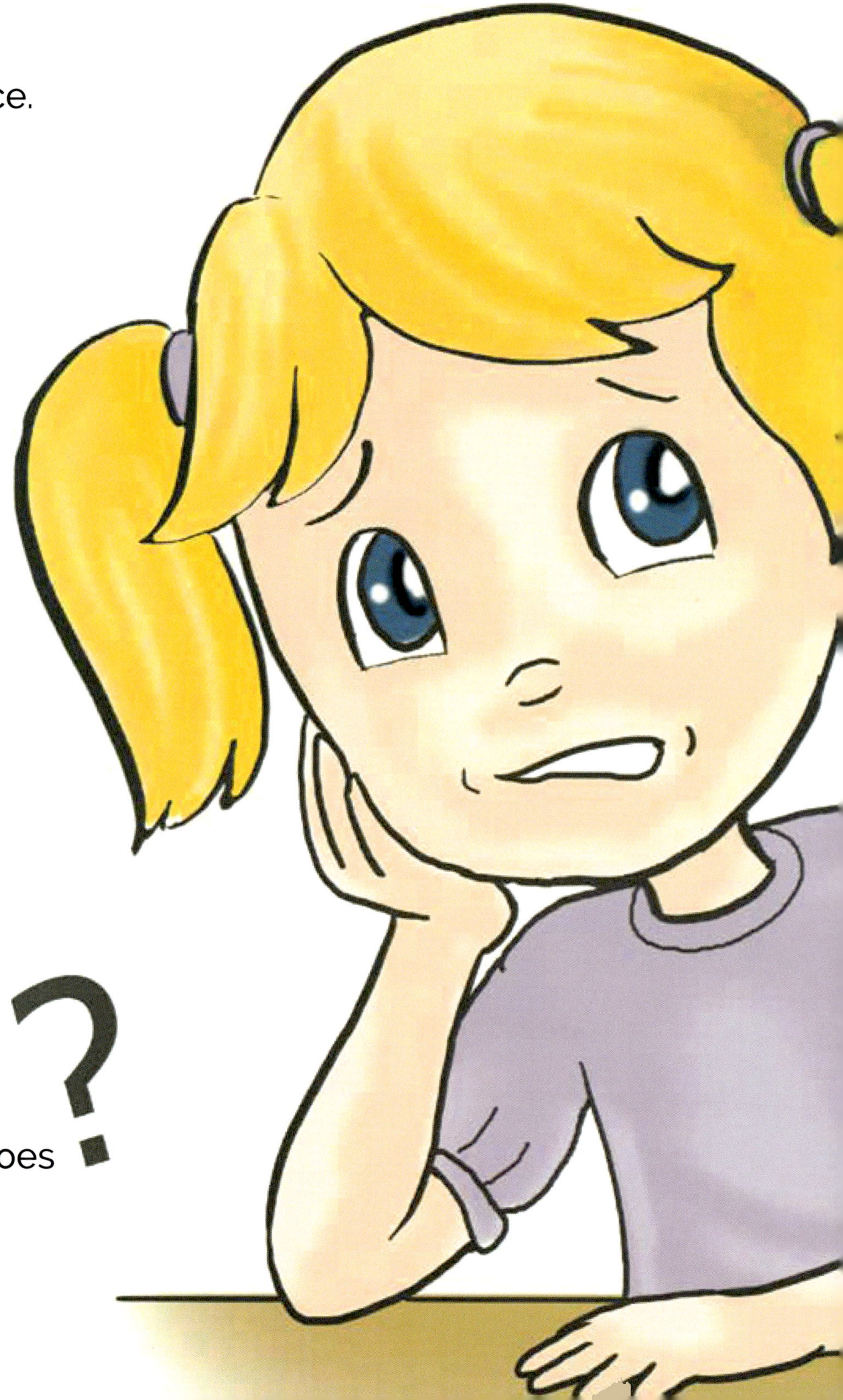

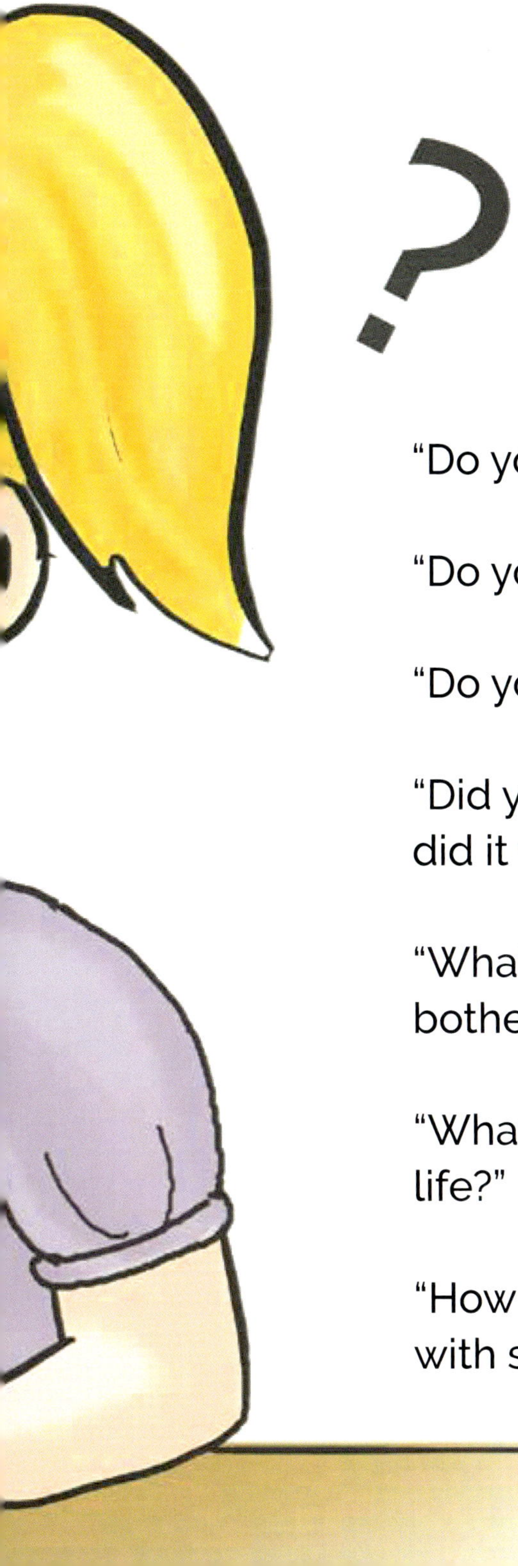

"When is the first time you saw or heard the one-legged pirate?"

"Do you like his company?"

"Do you want the voice to stay or go away?"

"Do you want to do away with the one-legged pirate?"

"Did you ever try to get rid of him? What did you try and how well did it work?"

"What would it be like if the pirate's voice was manageable and not bothersome?"

"What would it be like if the one-legged pirate remained in your life?"

"How do you feel about sharing all these details about the pirate with someone?"

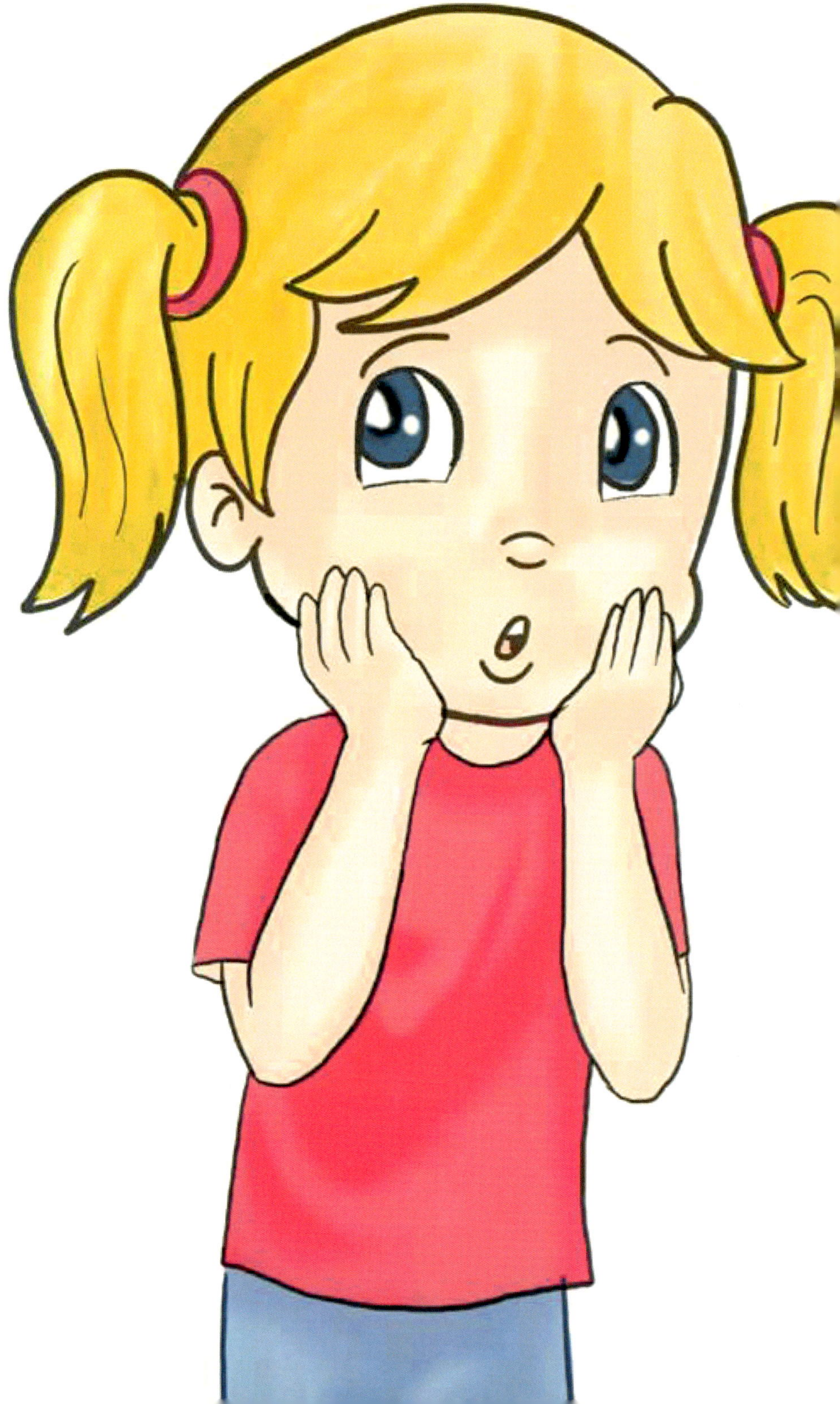

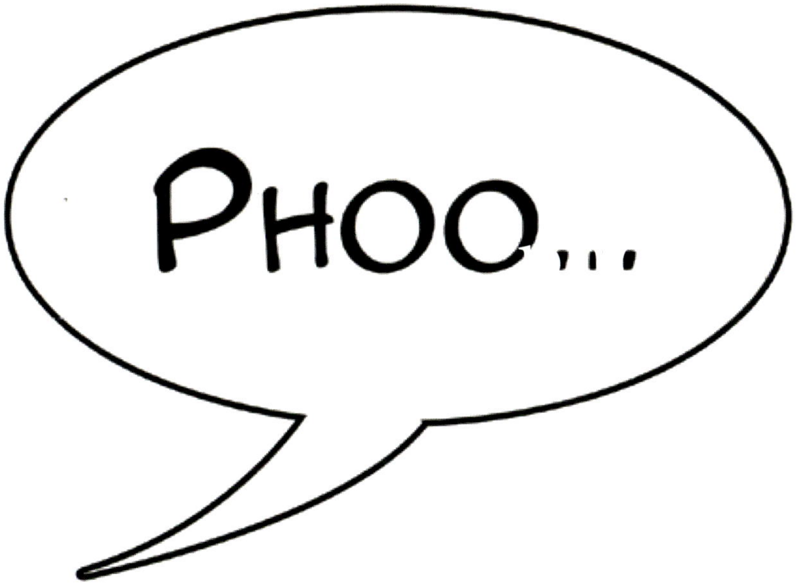

Phoo! Did I feel **overwhelmed** by all those questions!

But I really wanted Amy to understand what was going on with me.

So over the next few weeks, I slowly answered all her questions as best as I could.

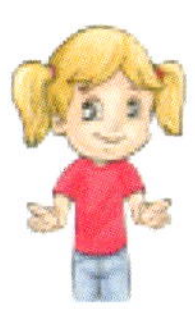

Have you ever been asked lots of really hard questions?
How did you feel?

The one-legged pirate pestered me every day.

He liked to confuse me when I had to think and focus or answer test questions at school. He would bully me into picking the wrong answers and then make fun of me.

"Only dumb people would pick that answer," he'd say in his gruff voice.

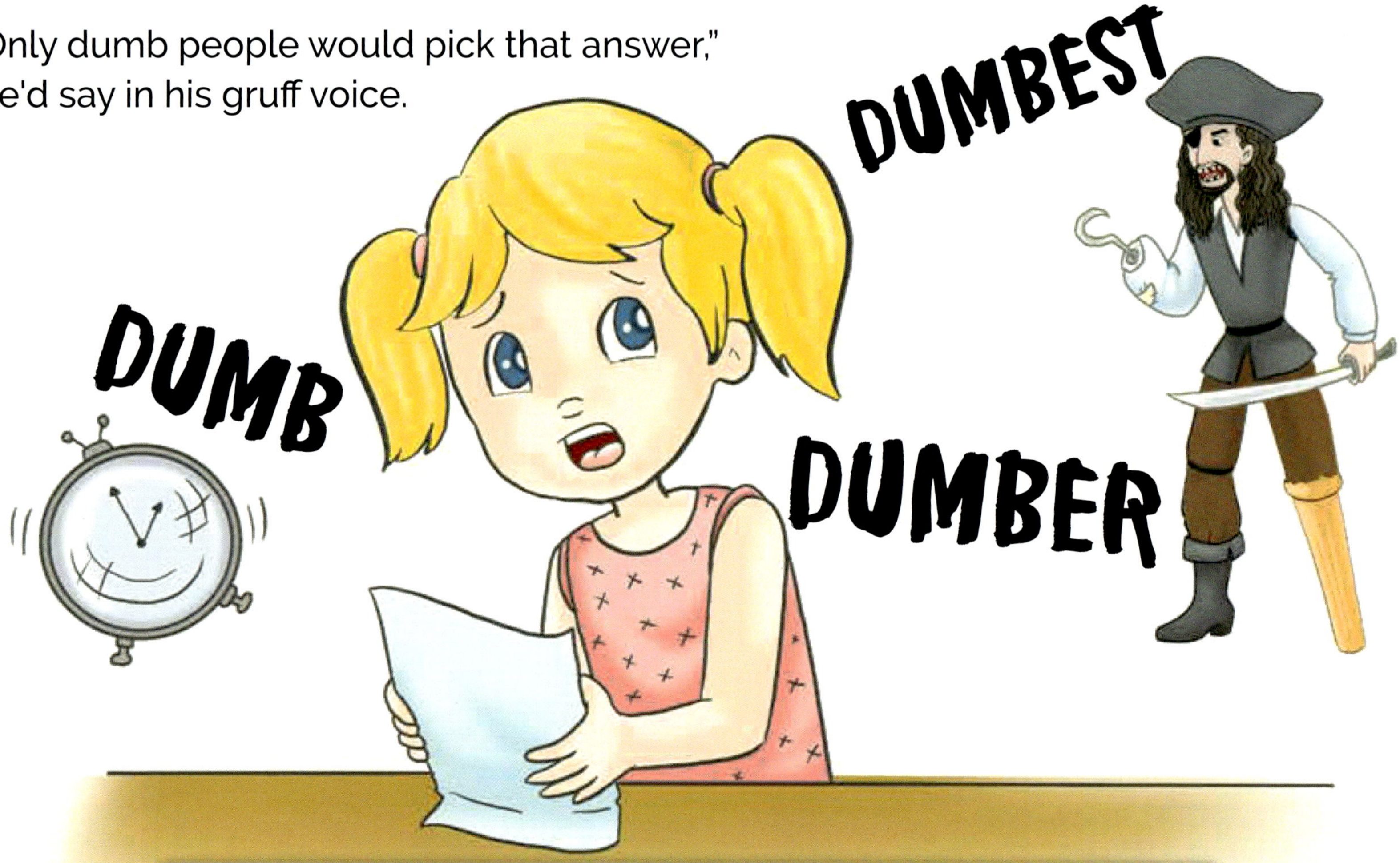

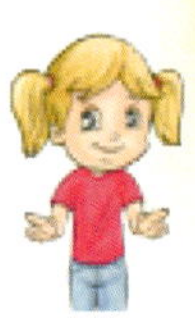

Do you think what the one-legged pirate did was mean?

When I had to make a decision, like whether to make a right or a left turn to get somewhere or whether I should wear shorts or pants to the park, the one-legged pirate would interrupt me. He chattered non-stop and made it hard for me to hear my own thoughts.

A lot of the time I felt like I was going to lose my mind!

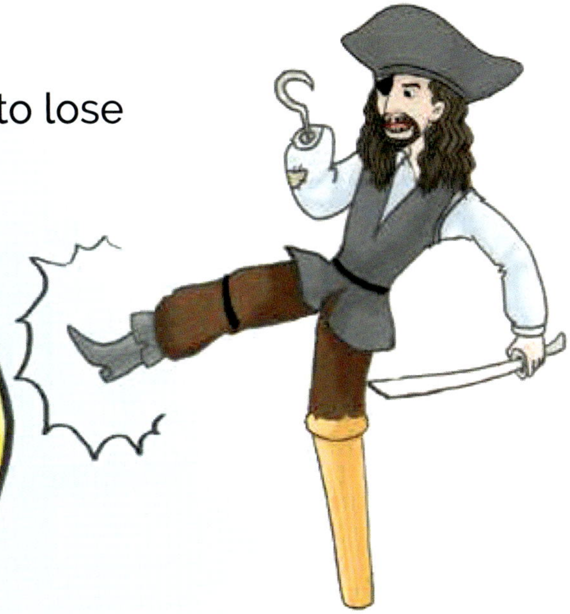

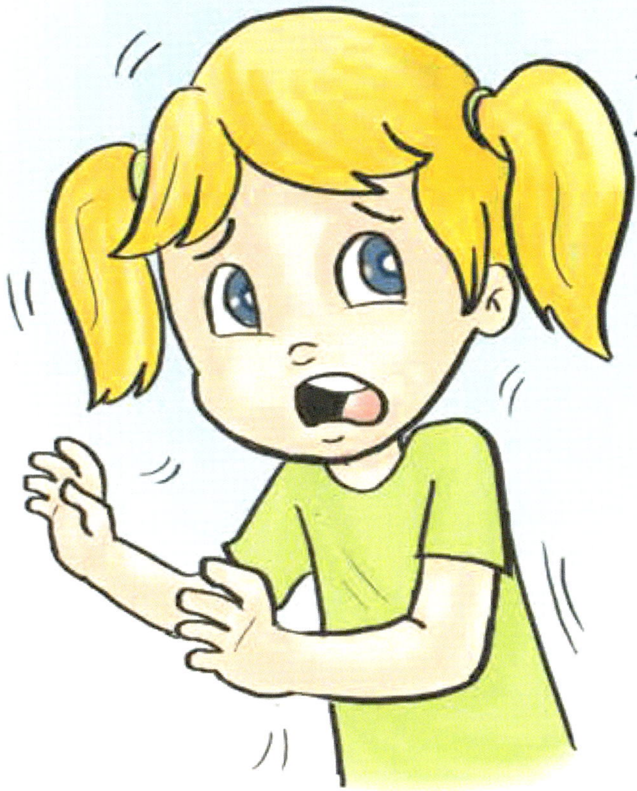

Though he came around every day, I never knew when he would show up or when he would leave.

To make matters worse, for no reason at all, he'd sometimes threaten to kick and hit me.

He was definitely a **PAIN**!

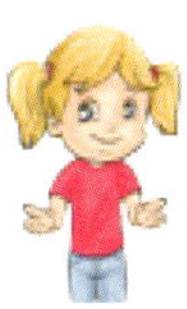

When does your voice come around?
What does he/she/it do or say?

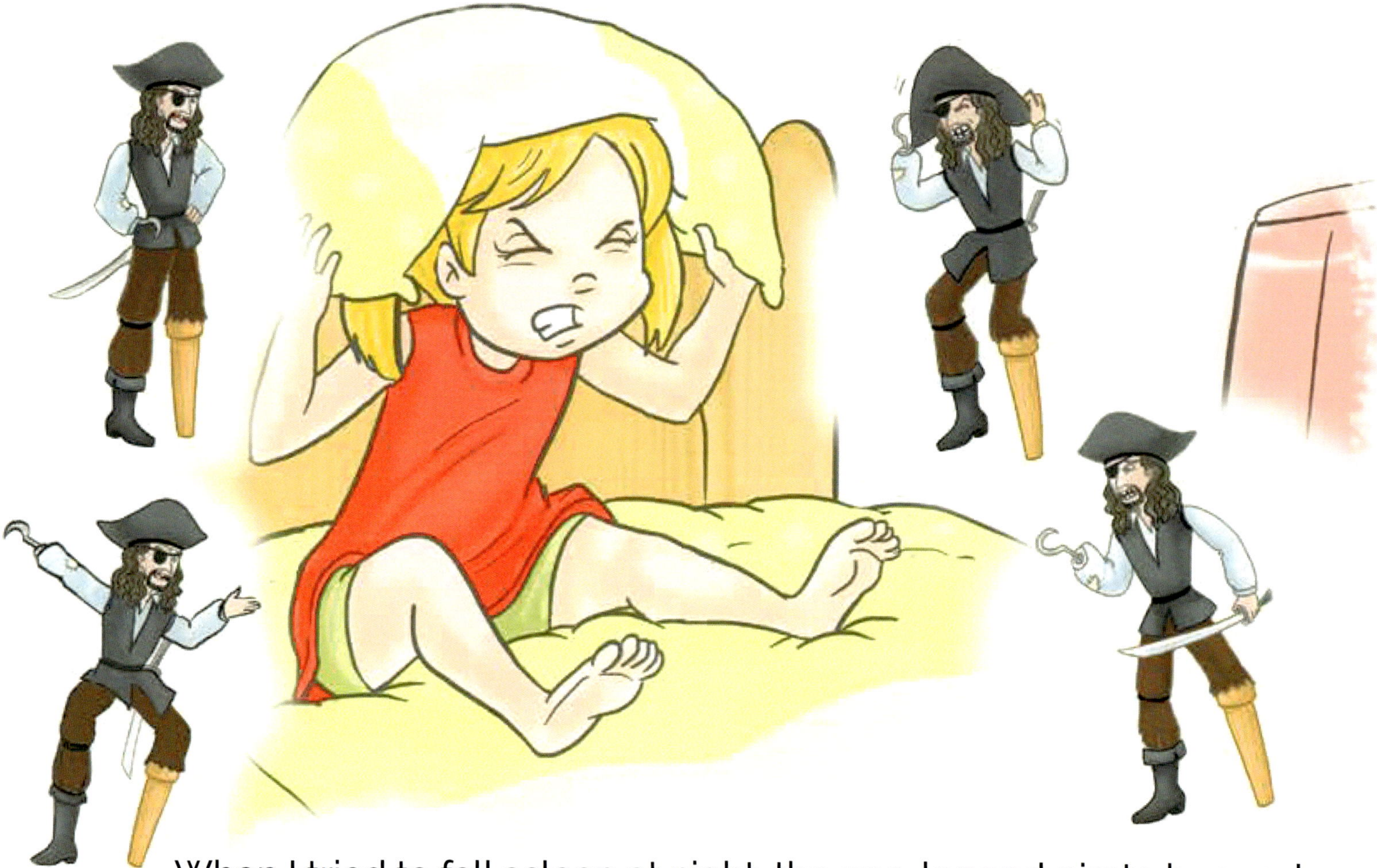

When I tried to fall asleep at night, the one-legged pirate bugged me by singing pirate songs as **LOUDLY** as he could.

I tried telling him to **STOP**.

I covered my ears with my hands. I put a pillow between him and me so I didn't have to look at him.

Nothing worked! I ran out of hope.

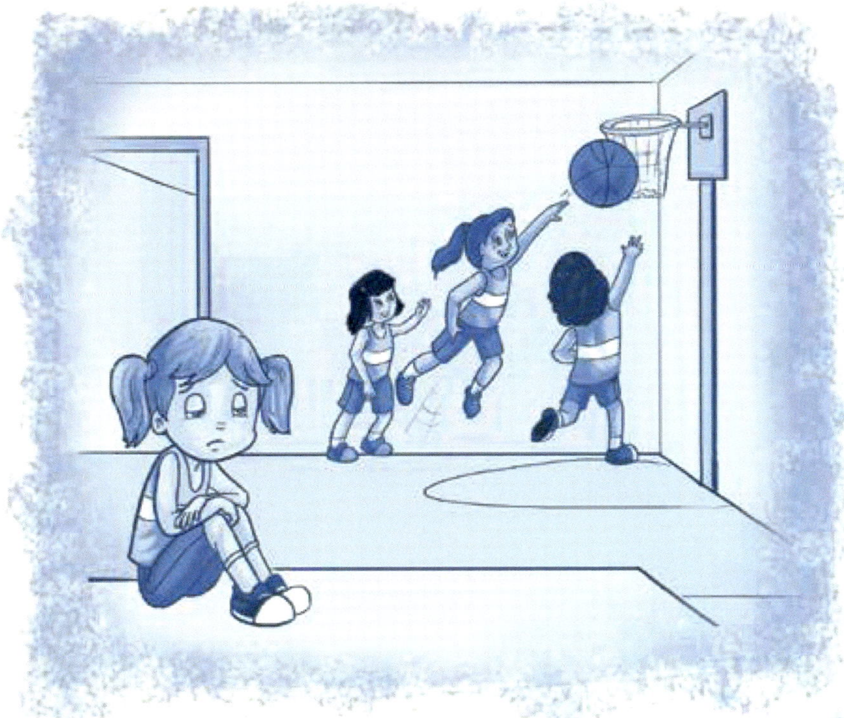

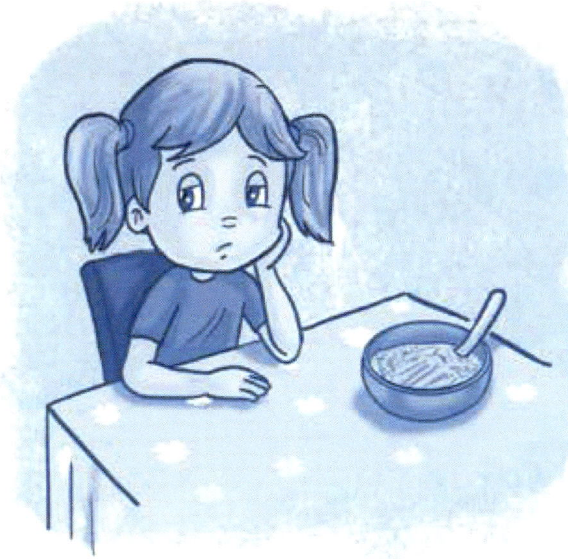

It seemed like none of the other kids at school had this problem.

I felt so sad so much of the time that I didn't feel like eating, playing, sleeping, talking to anyone, or doing my homework.

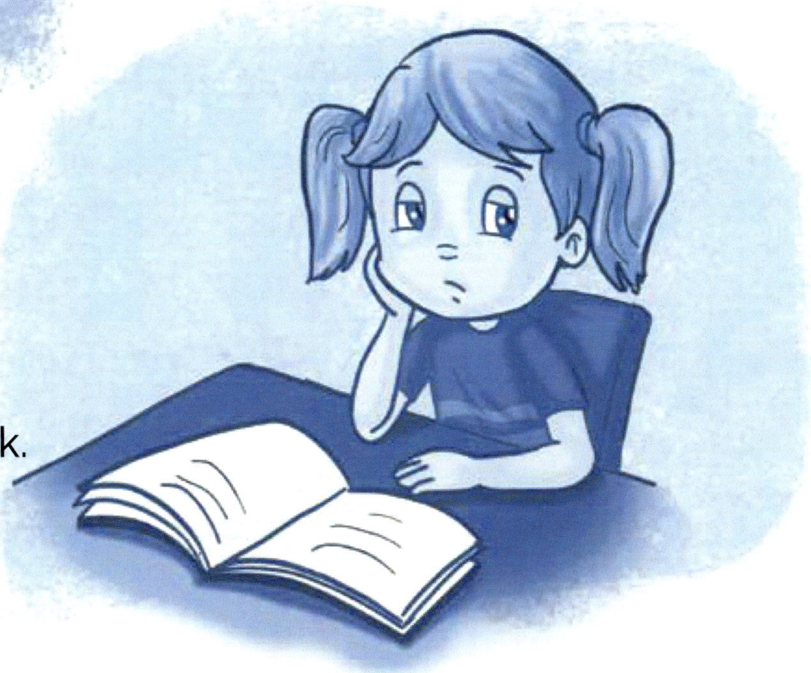

Sometimes I felt so terrible, I cried.

I wanted him out of my life!

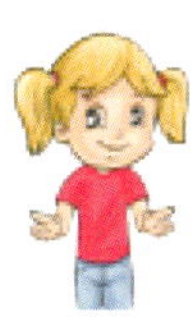

Does your voice bother you?
Would you like to keep your voice or prefer if it went away?

After sharing everything with Amy, I still felt bad. "I bet Amy thinks I'm a **'WEIRDO'**," I thought to myself.

By this time, I really liked Amy and wanted her to like me too. So I gathered up my courage and softly asked,

"Do you think I'm weird because I hear a voice?"

As the words rolled out of my mouth, my throat felt like it had a basketball stuck in it and I couldn't breathe.

But, in a split second, Amy replied.

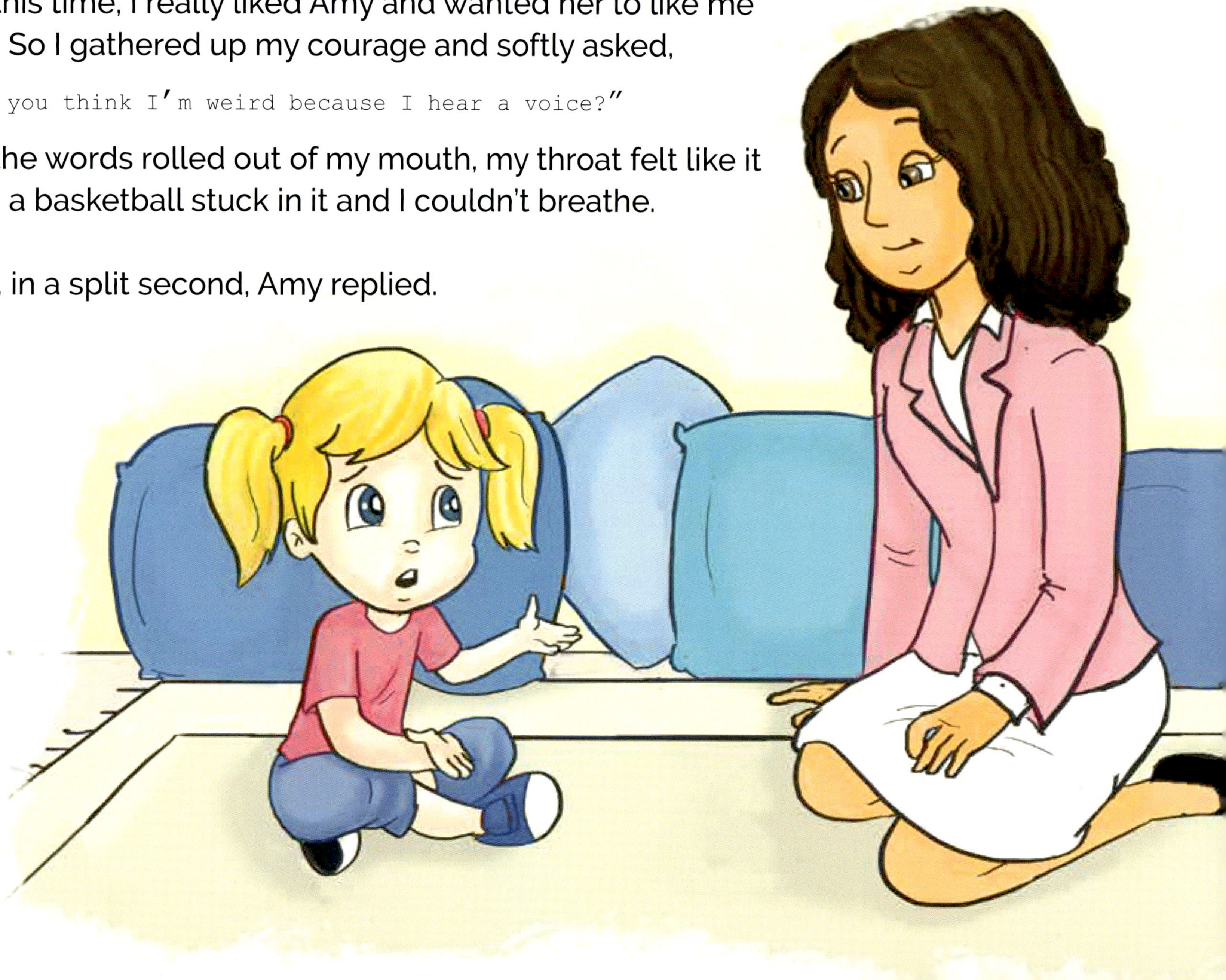

"No, certainly not, Susie! I think you are an awesome kid who hears voices.

Lots of kids and adults hear voices. Different people hear voices for different reasons. Often, people who hear voices fear them and don't talk about hearing voices. They feel uncomfortable and worry about what other people may think of them if they found out. They feel like they're the only ones on earth who hear voices.

Some people's voices stay for a short time and other people's voices stick around for a long time. Some voices can be enjoyable and entertaining and others may be uncomfortable, scary and embarrassing and you may feel like getting rid of them.

Voices can be a part of life. What is true is that once people learn about their voices, how they came about and figure out how to handle them, life can be good with or without voices.

It takes a lot of courage to take the first step to talk about hearing voices.

So that makes you a BRAVE kid, Susie, not a weird one." Amy said.

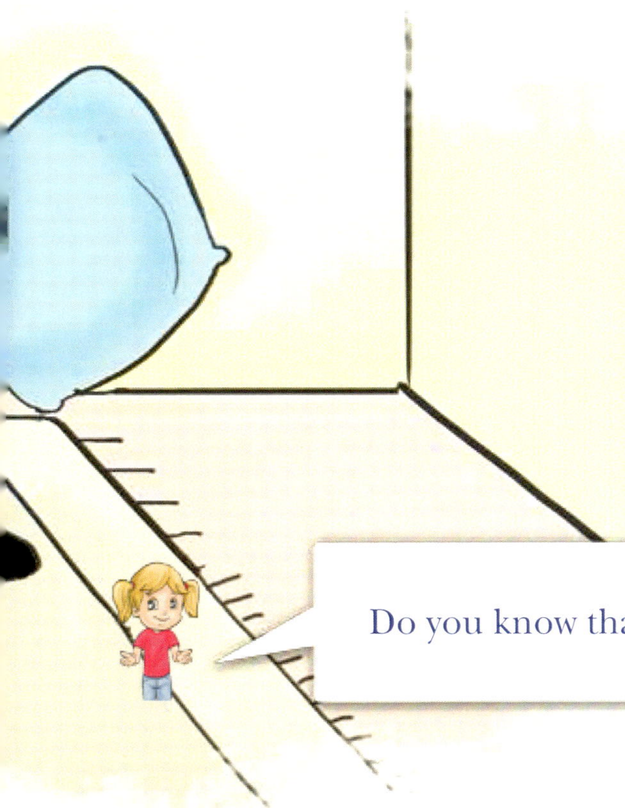

Do you know that there are many people out there who hear voices?

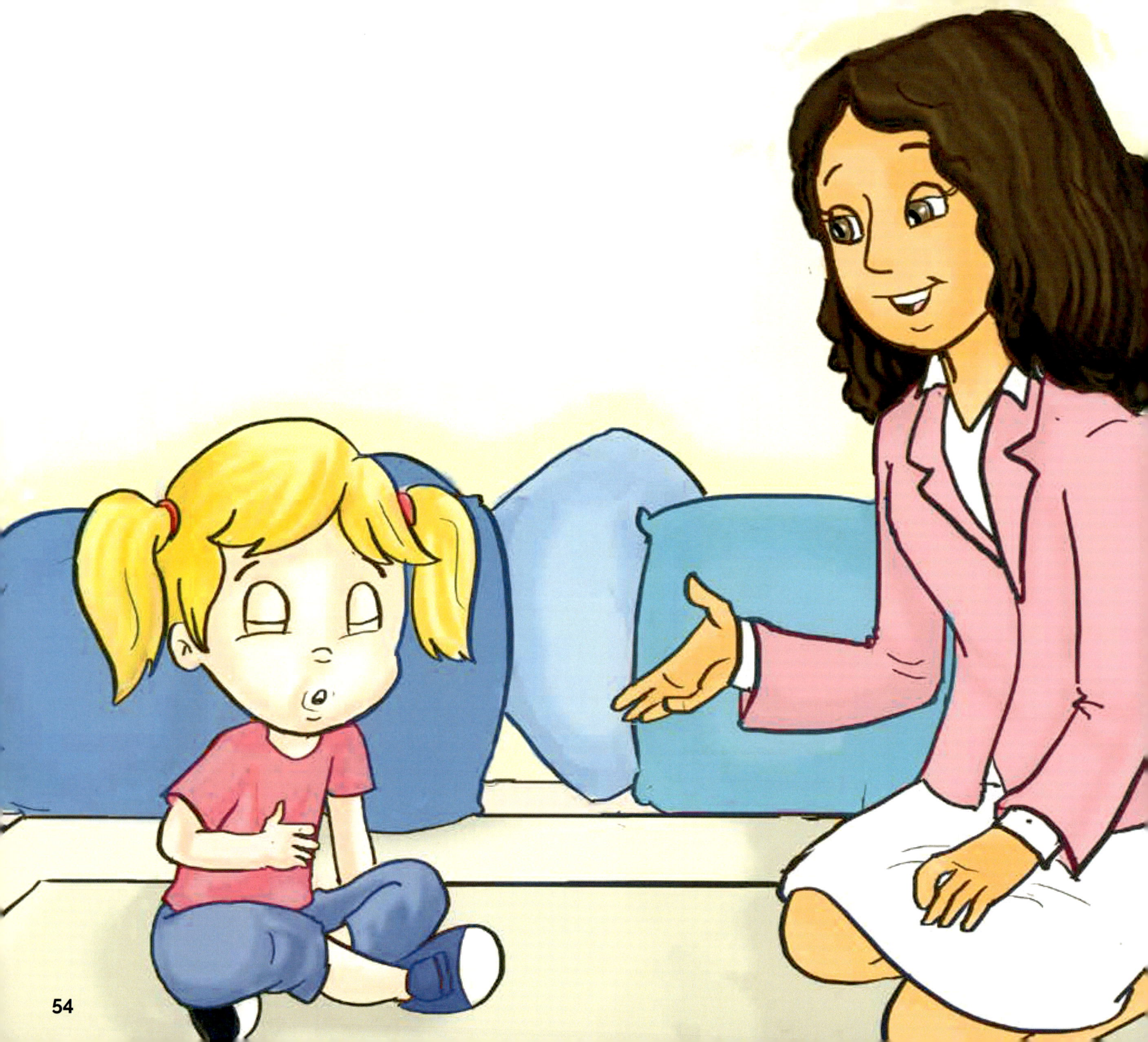

"Really, Amy?

I'm not **WEIRD**?

I'm not a **FREAK**?

I'm not **CRAZY**?

I'm not the only one? I'm not the only one who hears voices?

And voices can be managed?

People live with voices?" I asked, wide-eyed.

I was so **relieved** to hear that Amy didn't think I was weird!

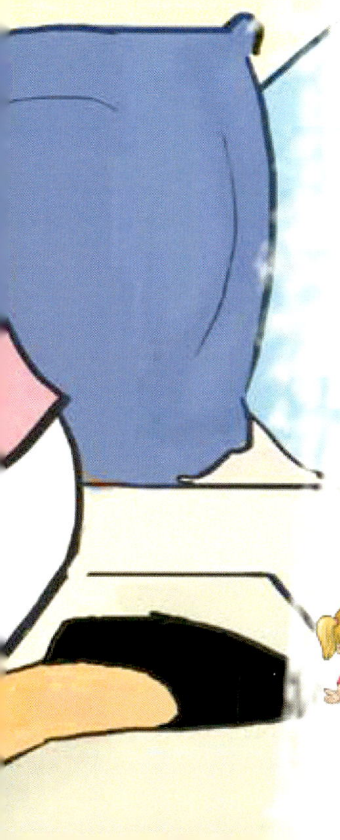

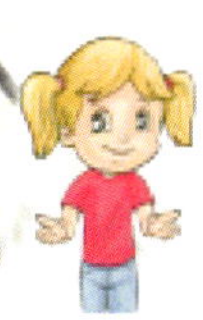

Are you **worried** that your counselor thinks you're **weird**?
Would you like to ask him/her what he/she thinks of you?
Go ahead and ask. I'll wait.

You know what?

Amy's right!

I'm not the only one. There are many other kids who hear voices.

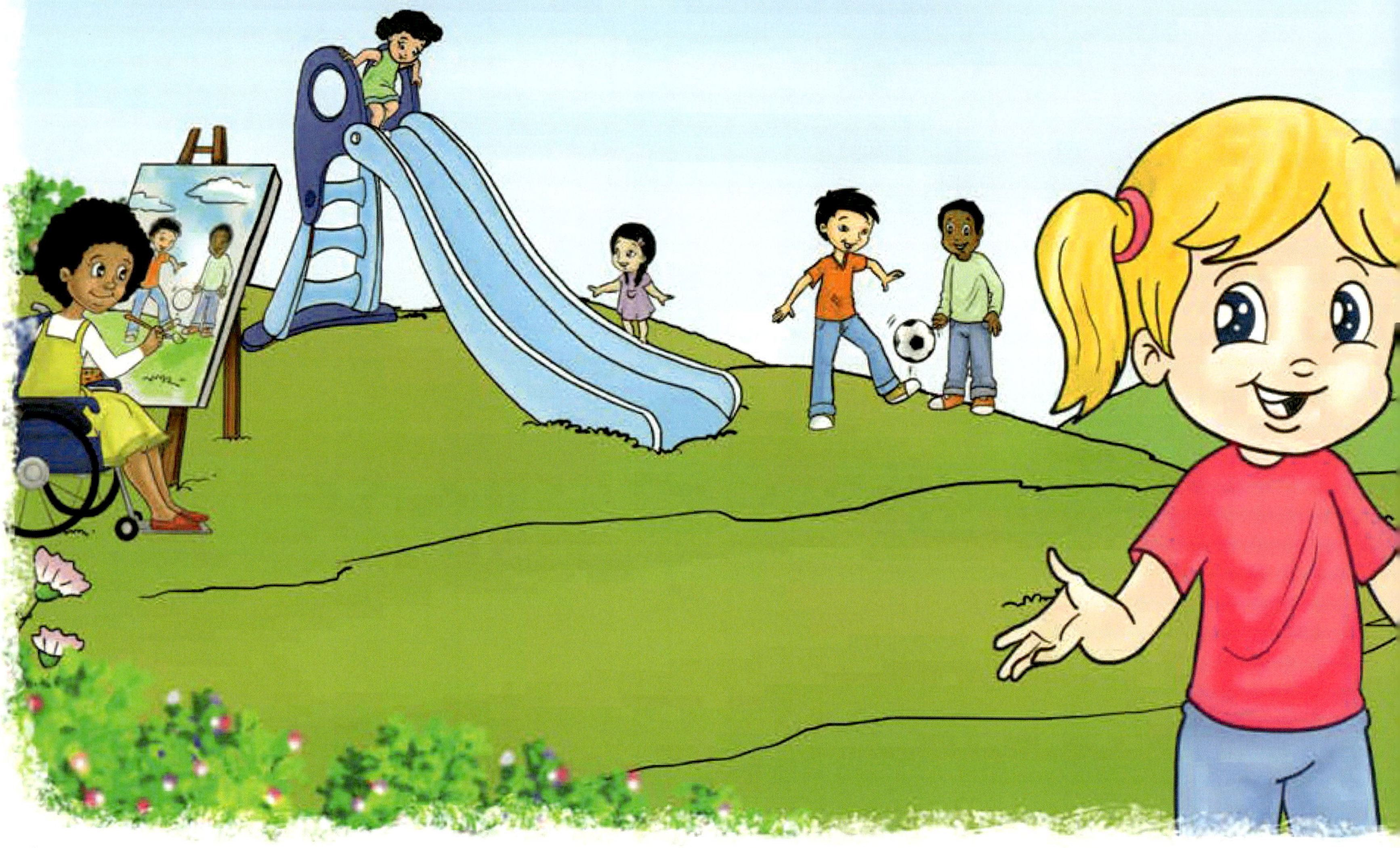

Would you like to know some of their stories?

If **yes,** read on.

If **no,** please **go to Chapter 6.**

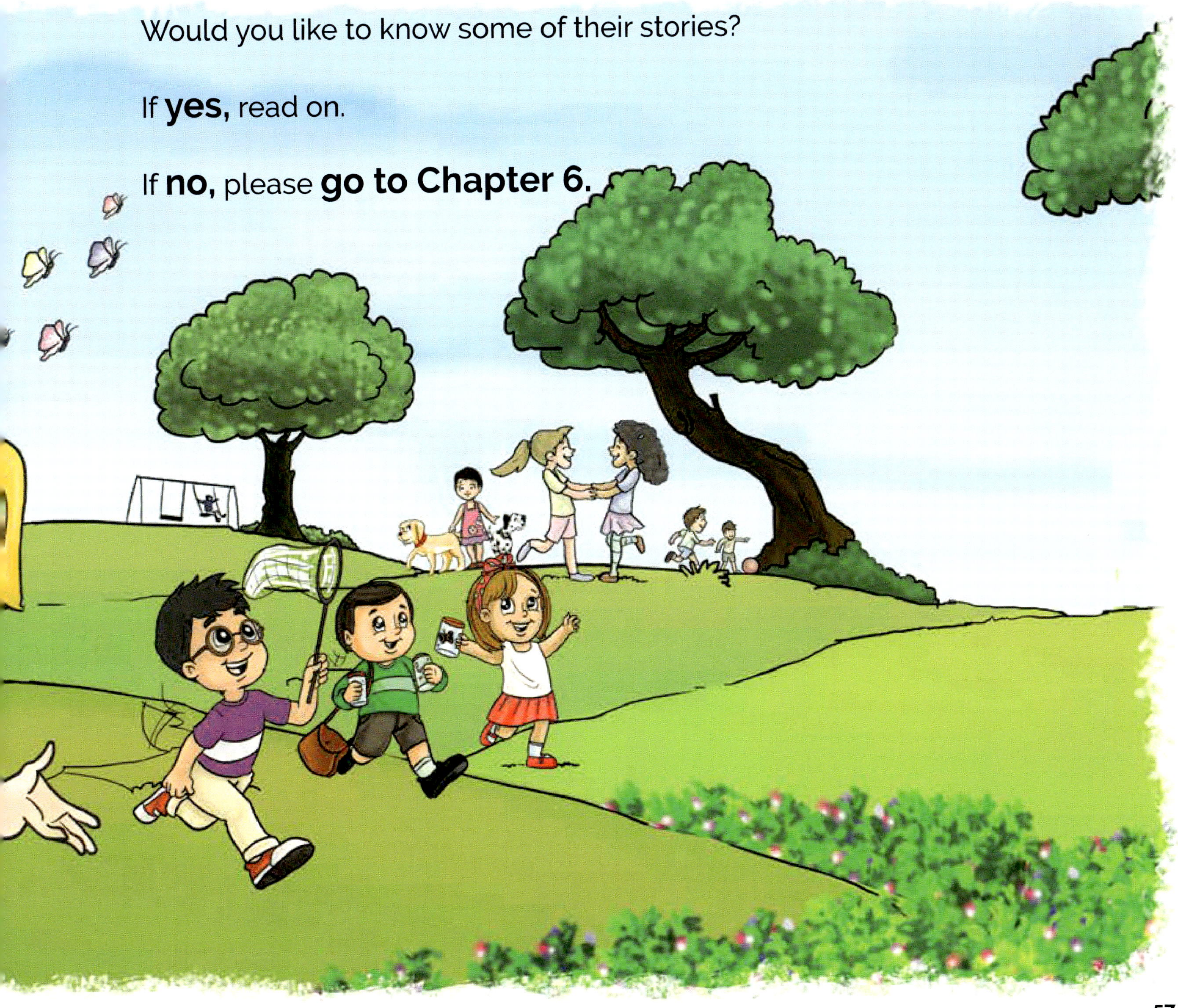

Chapter Two

Cackling Witch, Hissing Dragon

Meet Carlos.

Ever since his parents got a divorce less than a year ago, Carlos has been living with his father.

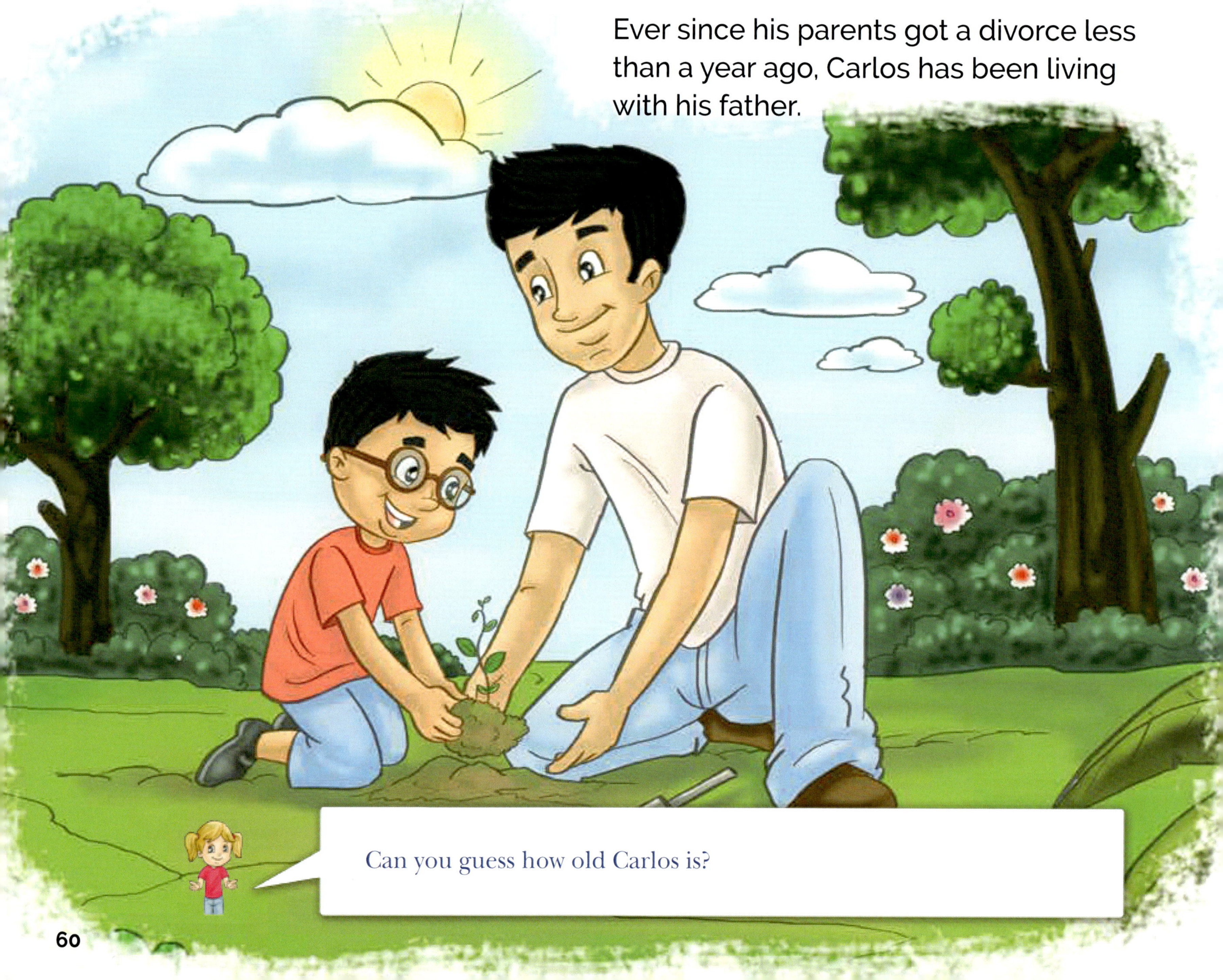

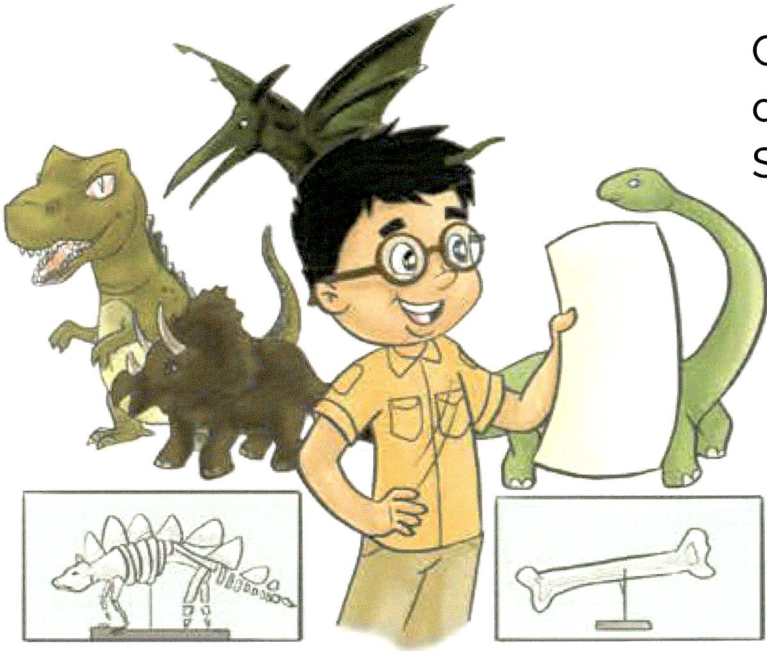

Carlos is 6 years old and is quite an expert on dinosaurs. He can tell you all about the Stegosaurus and Tyrannosaurus.

Can you guess what else Carlos likes?

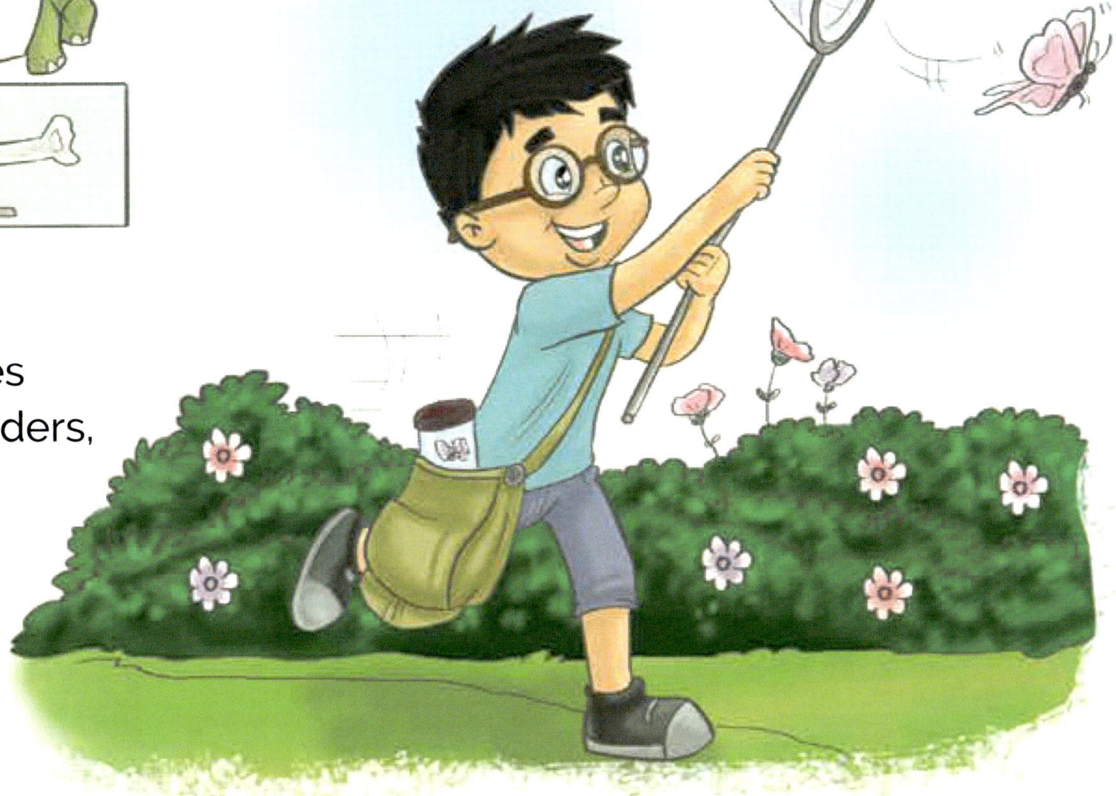

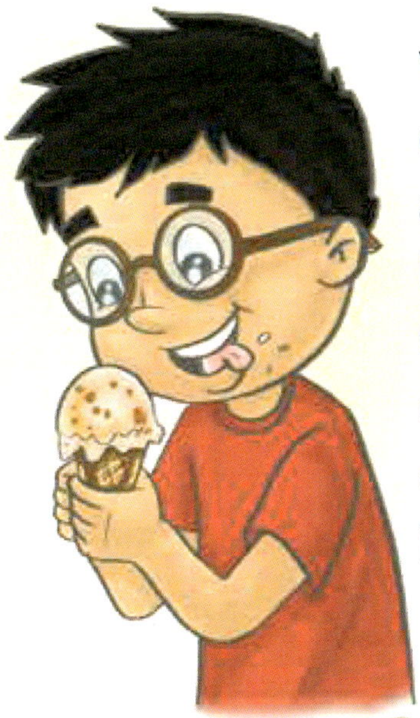

Well, besides catching spiders, ants and butterflies, Carlos likes chocolate chip ice cream!

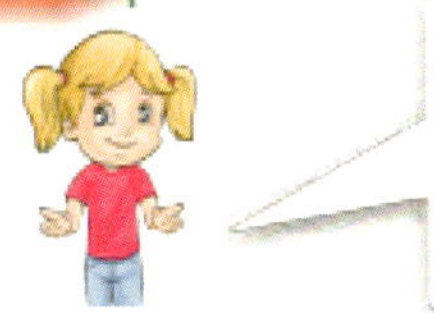

Do you like ice cream?
What is your favorite flavor?
What toppings do you like to have on yours?

For quite some time, Carlos heard and saw two voices.

One was a fire-blowing dragon that made hissing noises, and the other was a terrible witch who had a menacing laugh.

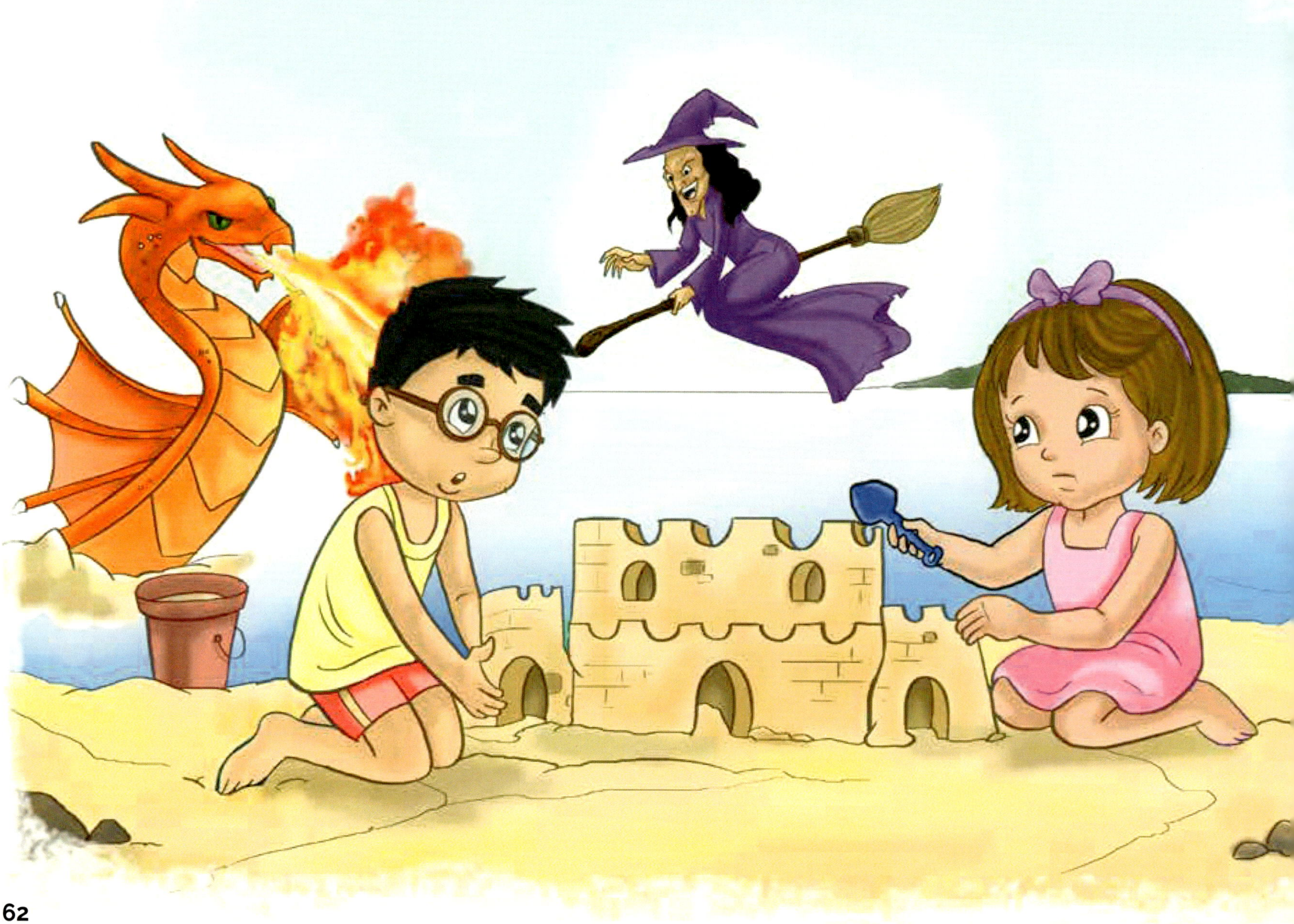

Carlos' voices usually appeared when he was playing with other kids.

When they first started bugging him, the sounds of the hissing dragon, his fire breathing and the witch's cackling were very soft and gentle. But the more Carlos tried to ignore them, the louder they got.

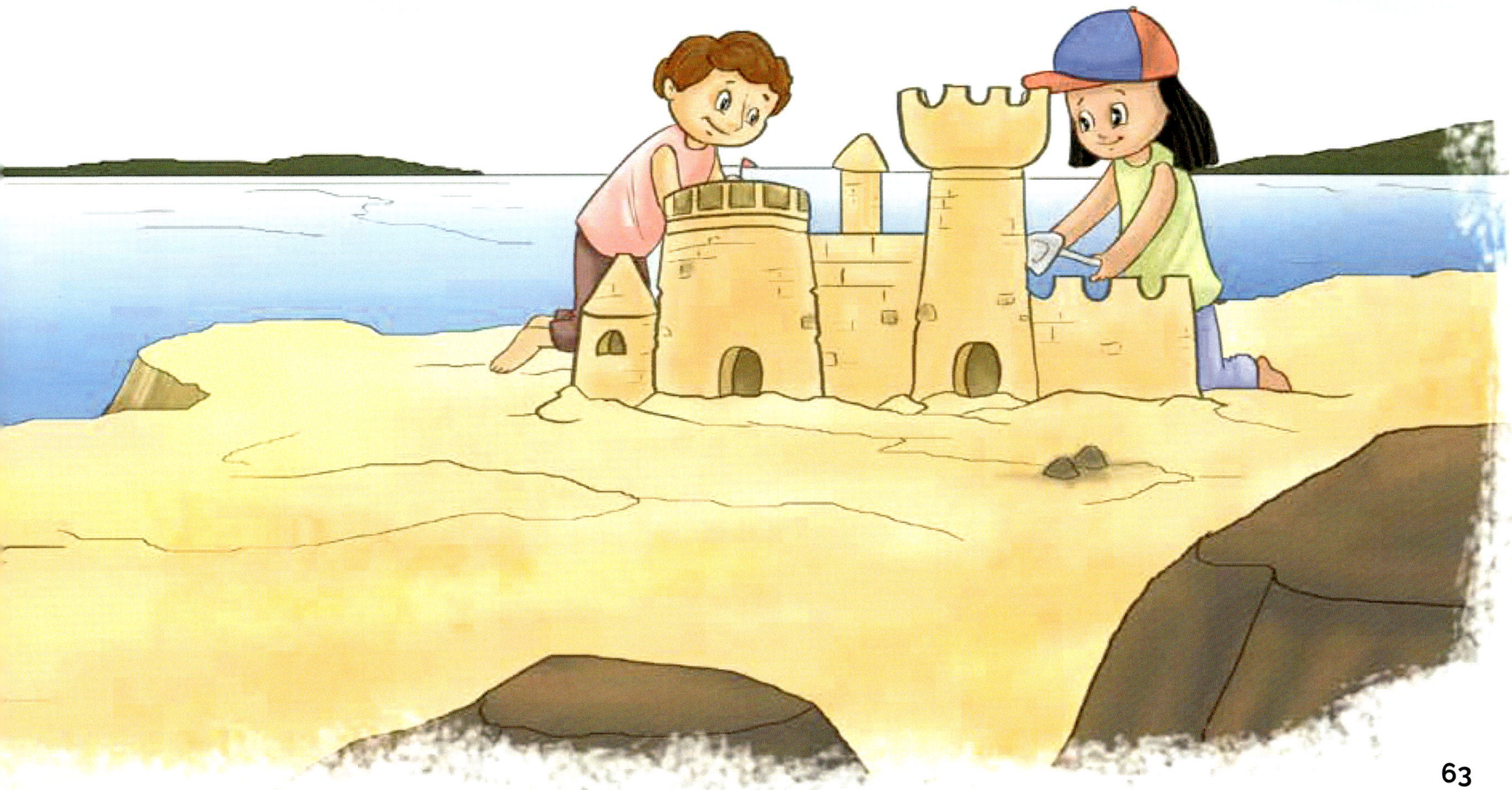

The dragon didn't talk, but you could tell he was boiling over with anger almost all of the time. While hiding behind bushes, he would blow fire at houses. His hot and bright yellow flames would sizzle homes to a cinder. At other times, his angry flames burned trees and even the clothes people were wearing.

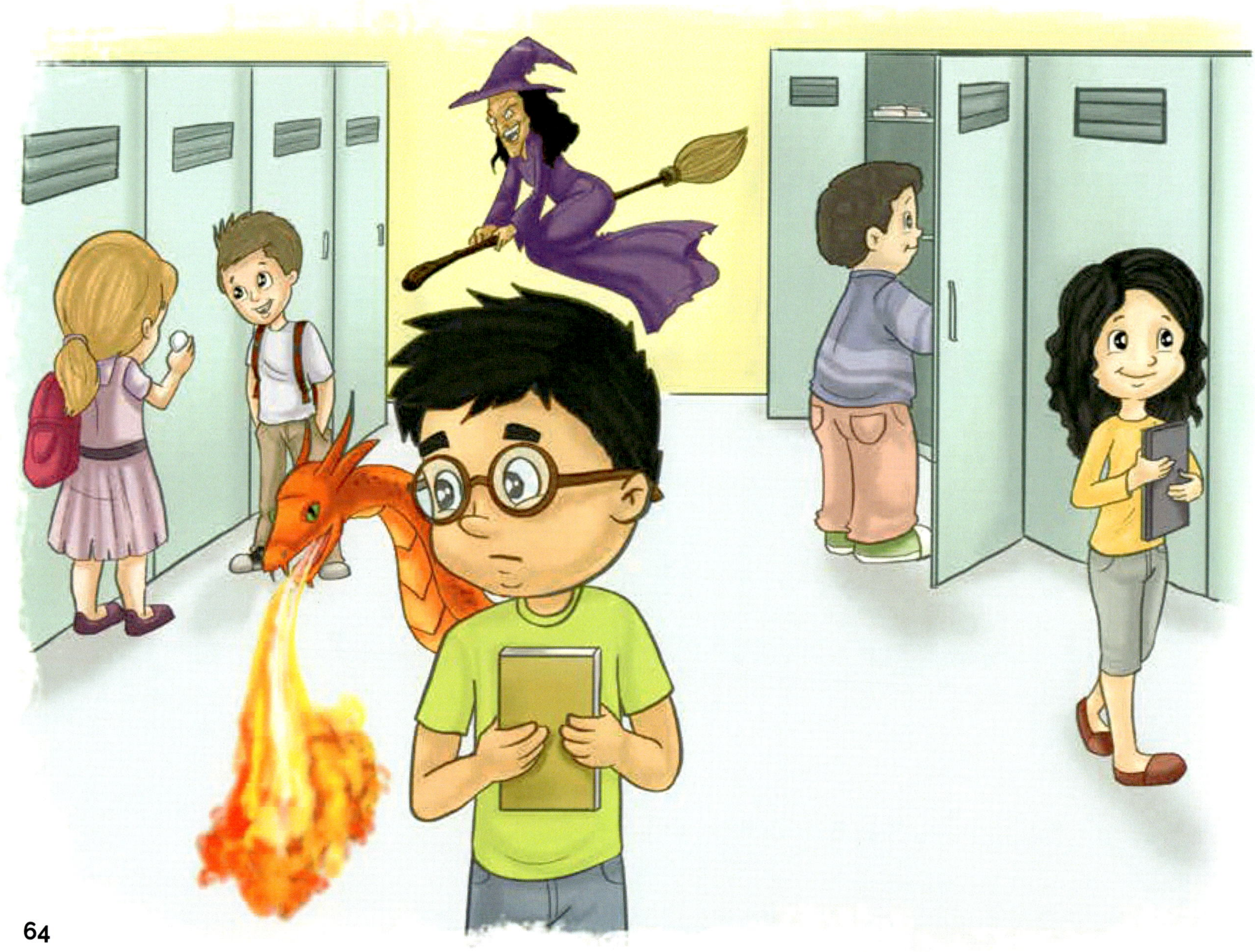

Unlike the dragon, the witch talked a lot.

She said lots of mean things like, "Everyone hates you! I hope you will die for all the terrible things you've done.

Die, Die, Die!!!

Hyah-hyah-hyah-hyah-hyah!"

The hissing dragon and cackling witch got so loud and **annoying** that Carlos could no longer have conversations with people without being distracted by them. Sometimes it felt like the witch and dragon ruled his life.

He felt powerless.

Carlos wanted to quiet the voices but didn't know how. He wanted to be in control of them, but it was too hard to do.

They would not behave.

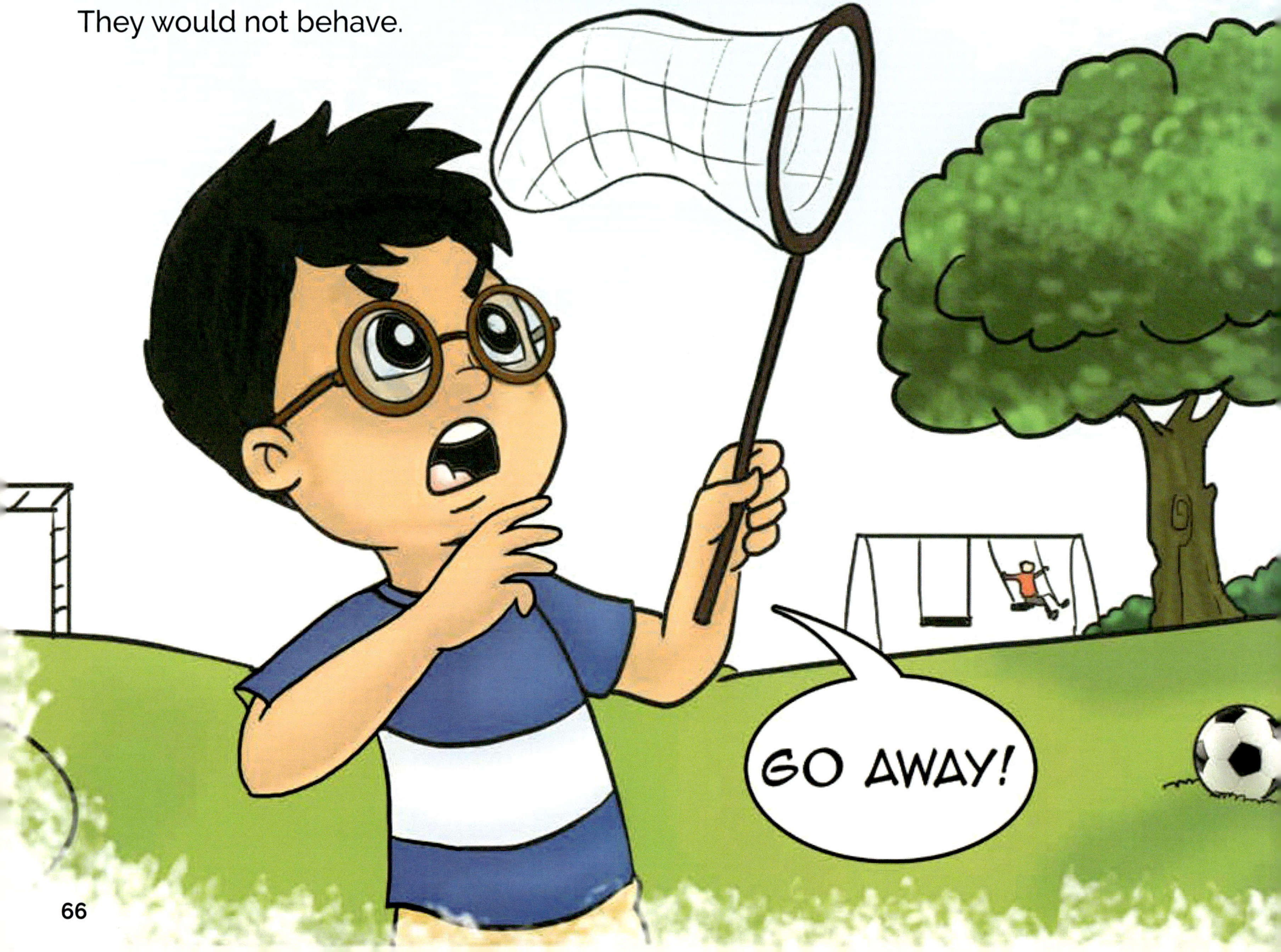

Sometimes he'd yell at them, and kids around him would be surprised. He'd feel **embarrassed.**

Afraid that people would think he was "nuts" and laugh at him, Carlos did not tell anyone about the hissing dragon or the cackling witch.

Slowly, he stopped being around others.

Carlos felt lost in his world of voices.

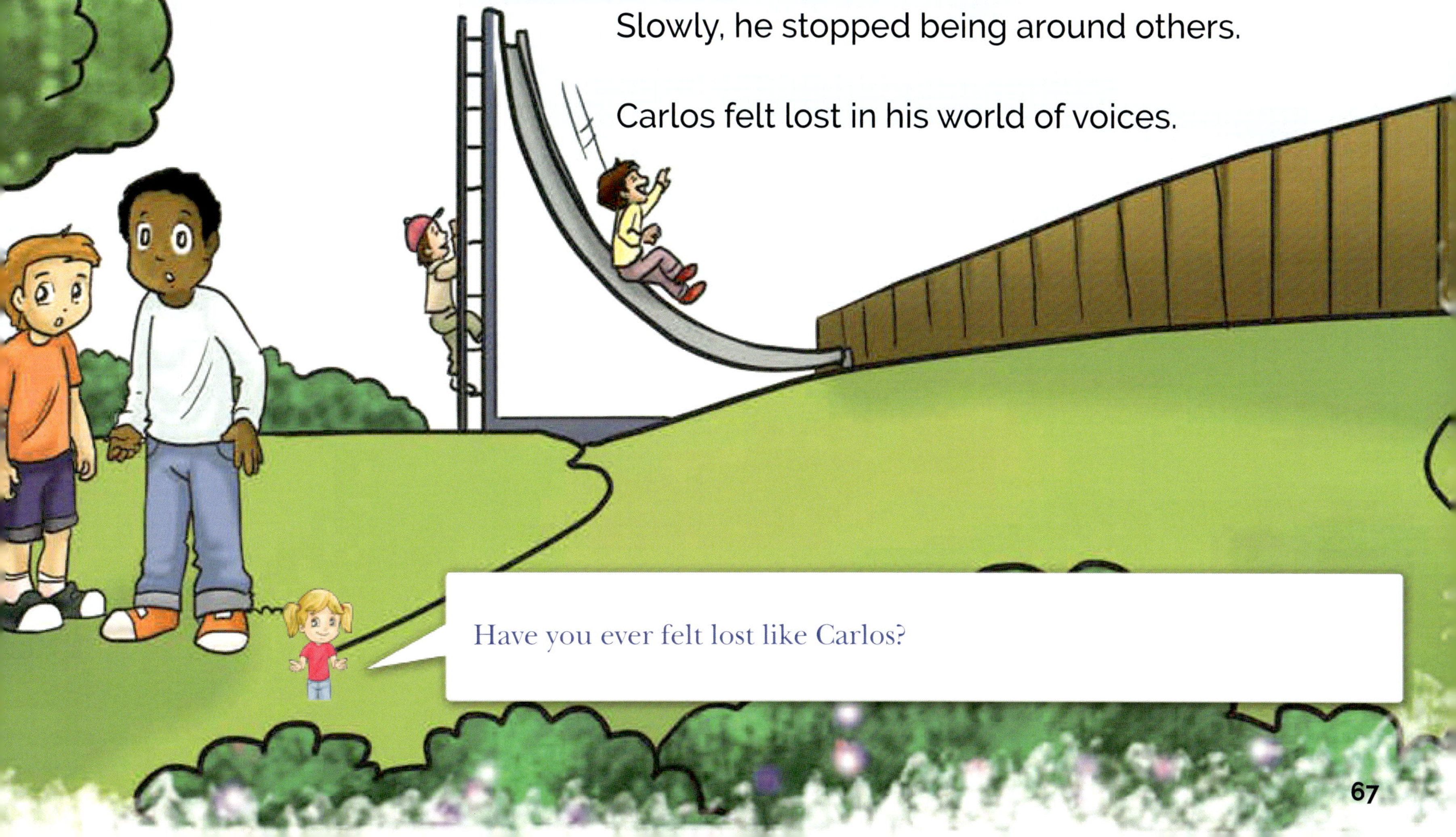

Some of the time, Carlos felt sad about the voices and wished someone would help him. But he never allowed himself to approach anyone about them. Often, it was hard for him to make sense of his confusing and mixed feelings. This made Carlos feel worse. He felt there was something wrong with him.

After some time, Carlos didn't feel like talking to anyone about the voices — or anything else for that matter. He longed for his life to be quiet and normal, like everyone else's.

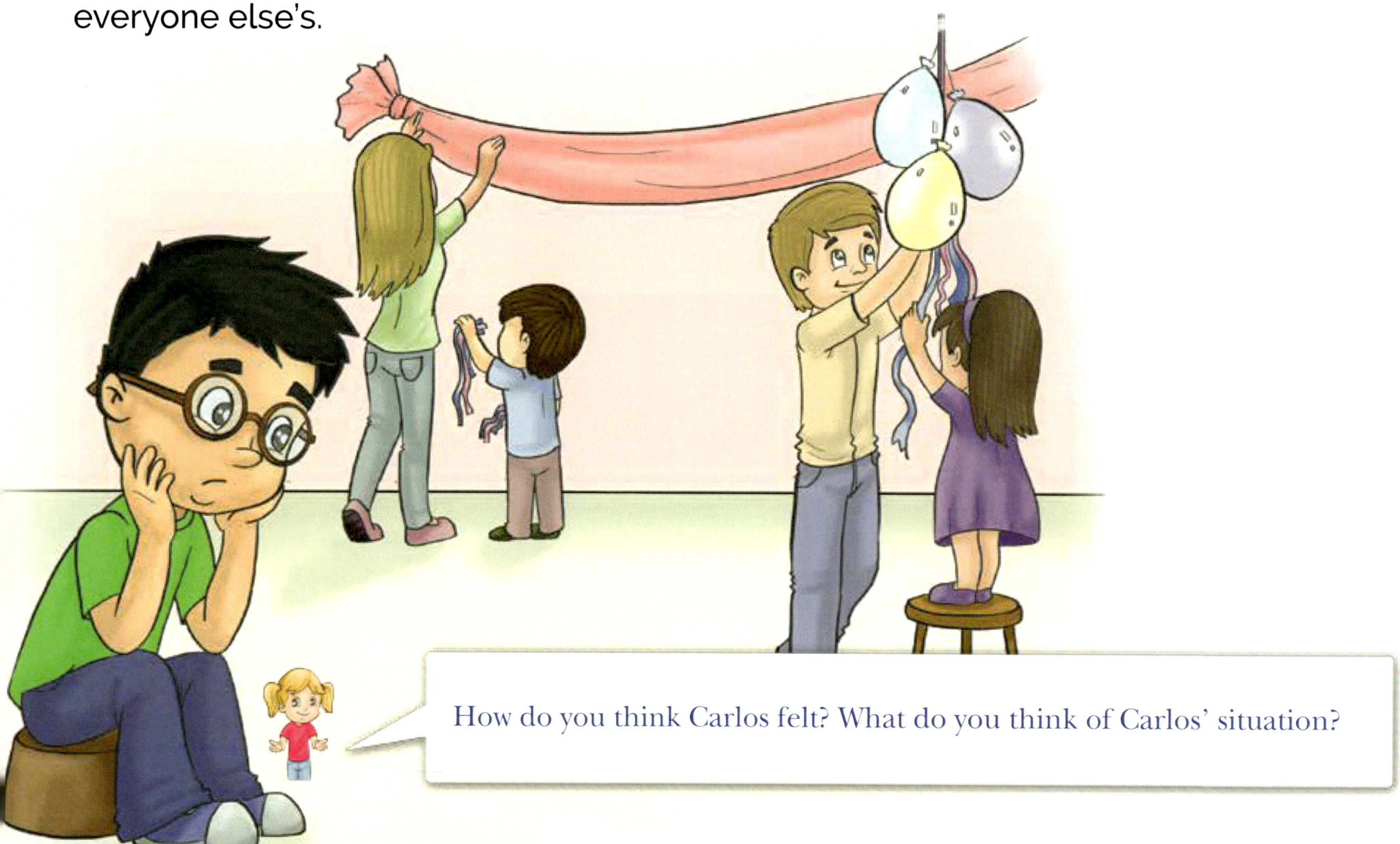
How do you think Carlos felt? What do you think of Carlos' situation?

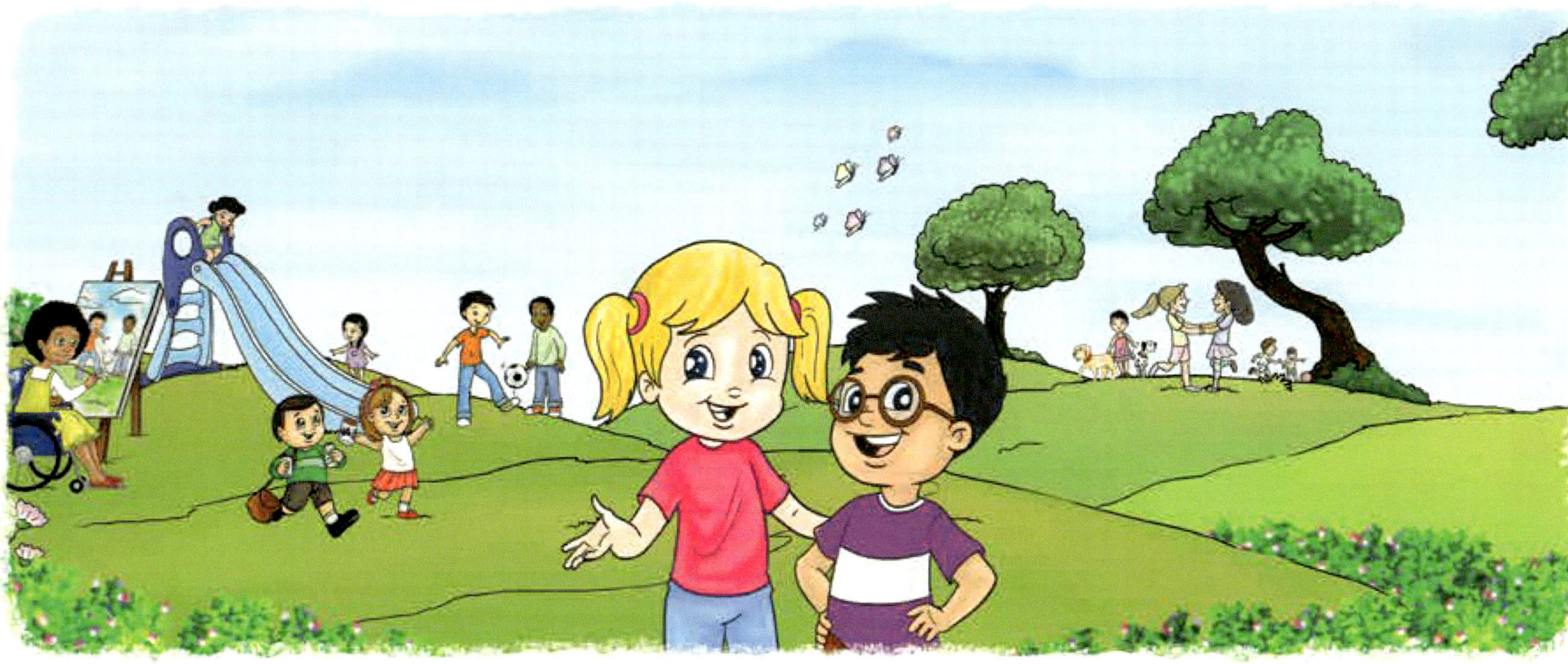

Just like me, Carlos thought he was the only kid on earth who struggled with voices.

He was surprised to know about the girl who heard more voices than he did!

Let me introduce you to her.

Read on if you would like to know **her story.**

If **no, skip** forward **to Chapter 6.**

Chapter Three

The Squabblers

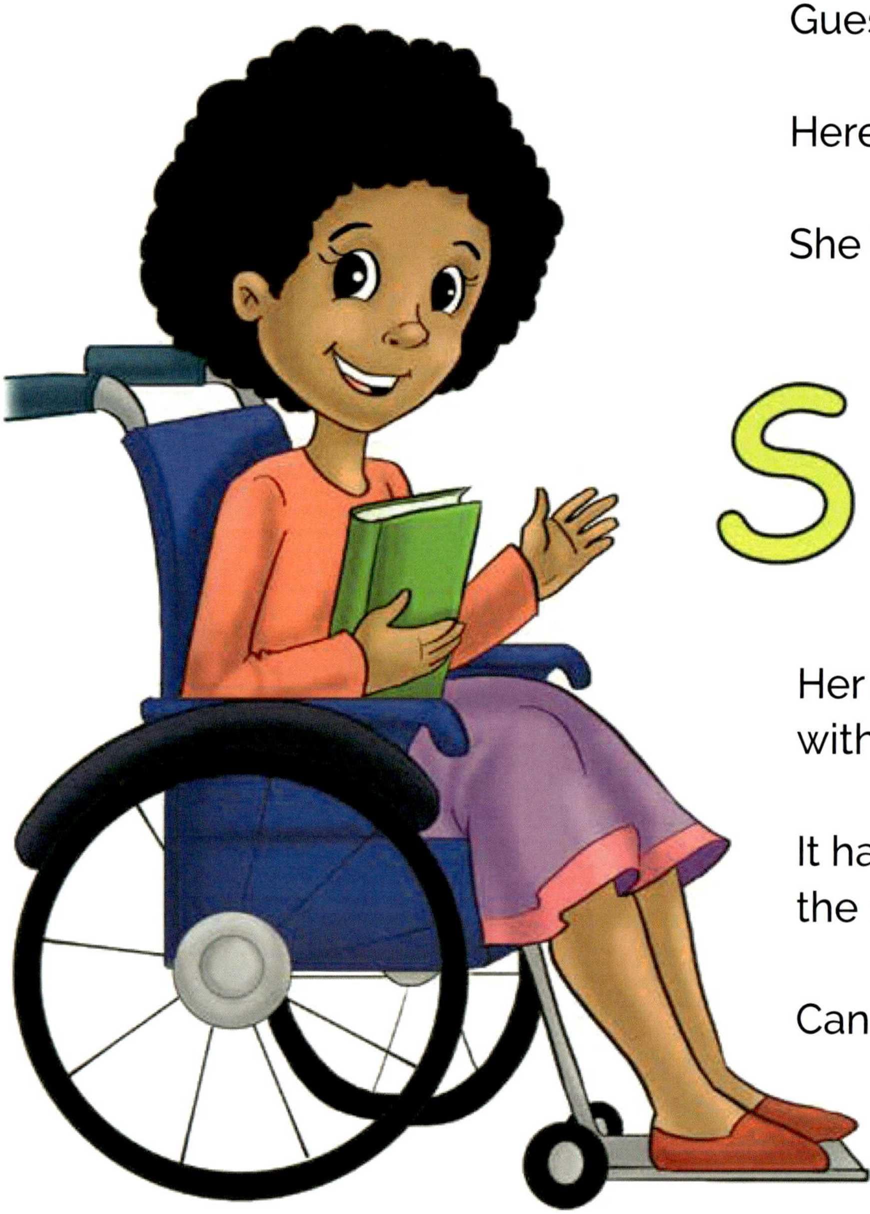

Guess who this is?

Here are some clues.

She is 15 years old.

S _ _ _ A

Her name starts with the letter S, ends with the letter A.

It has 5 letters in it, and rhymes with the name "Thelma".

Can you figure out her name?

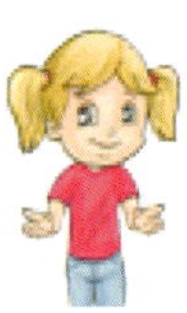

The name Selma can be a hard one to guess. Did you get it?

Selma paints beautifully and loves to go on fishing trips with her foster dad.

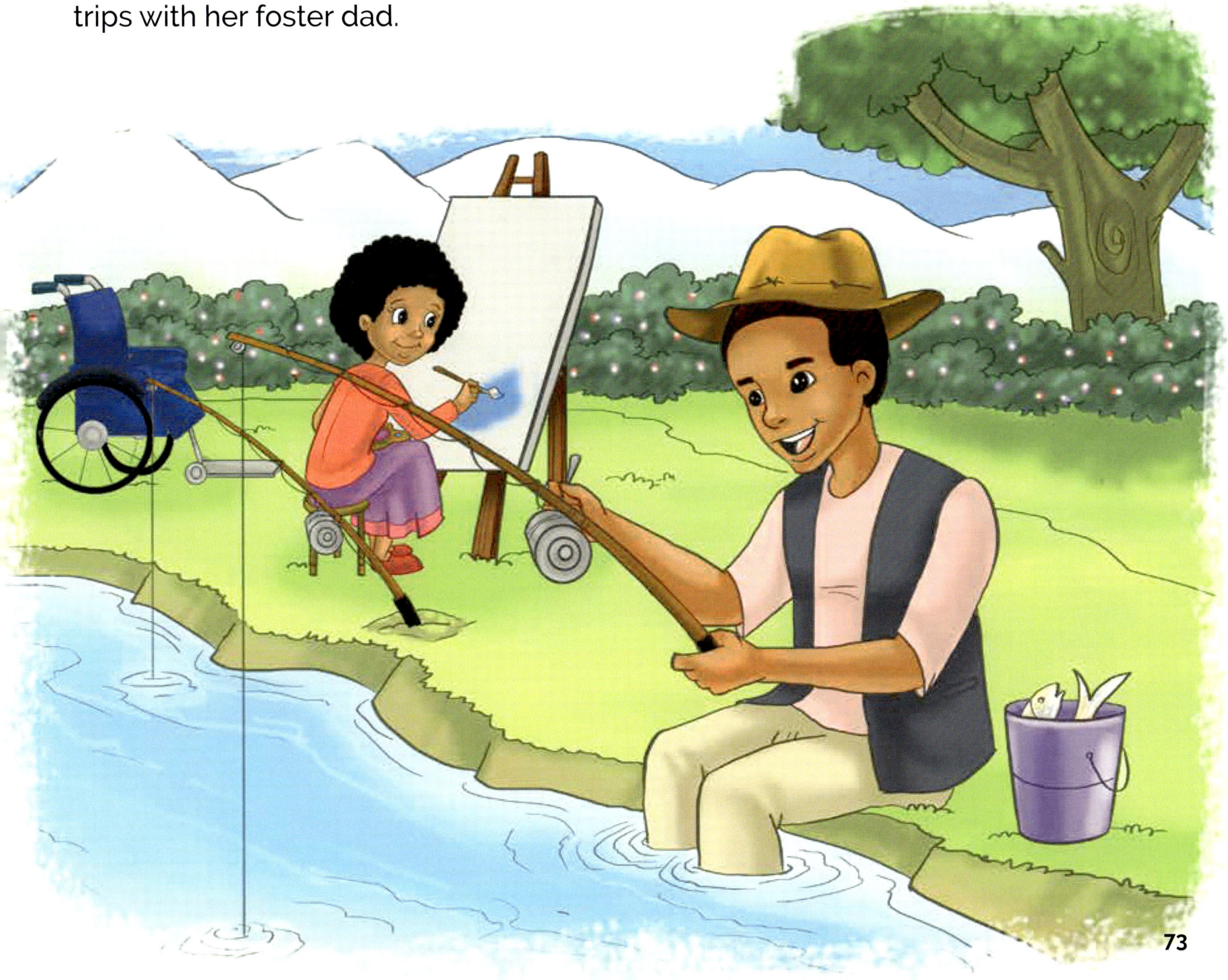

Being pretty shy, talking about the voices is really difficult for Selma.

However, she thinks it's important that kids like you know you are not the only ones who hear voices.

So, here goes.

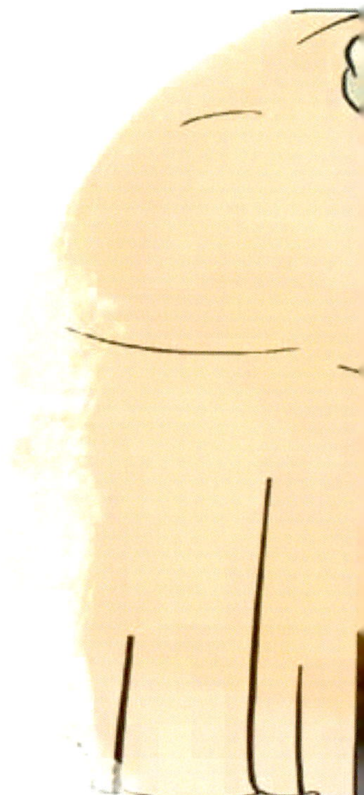

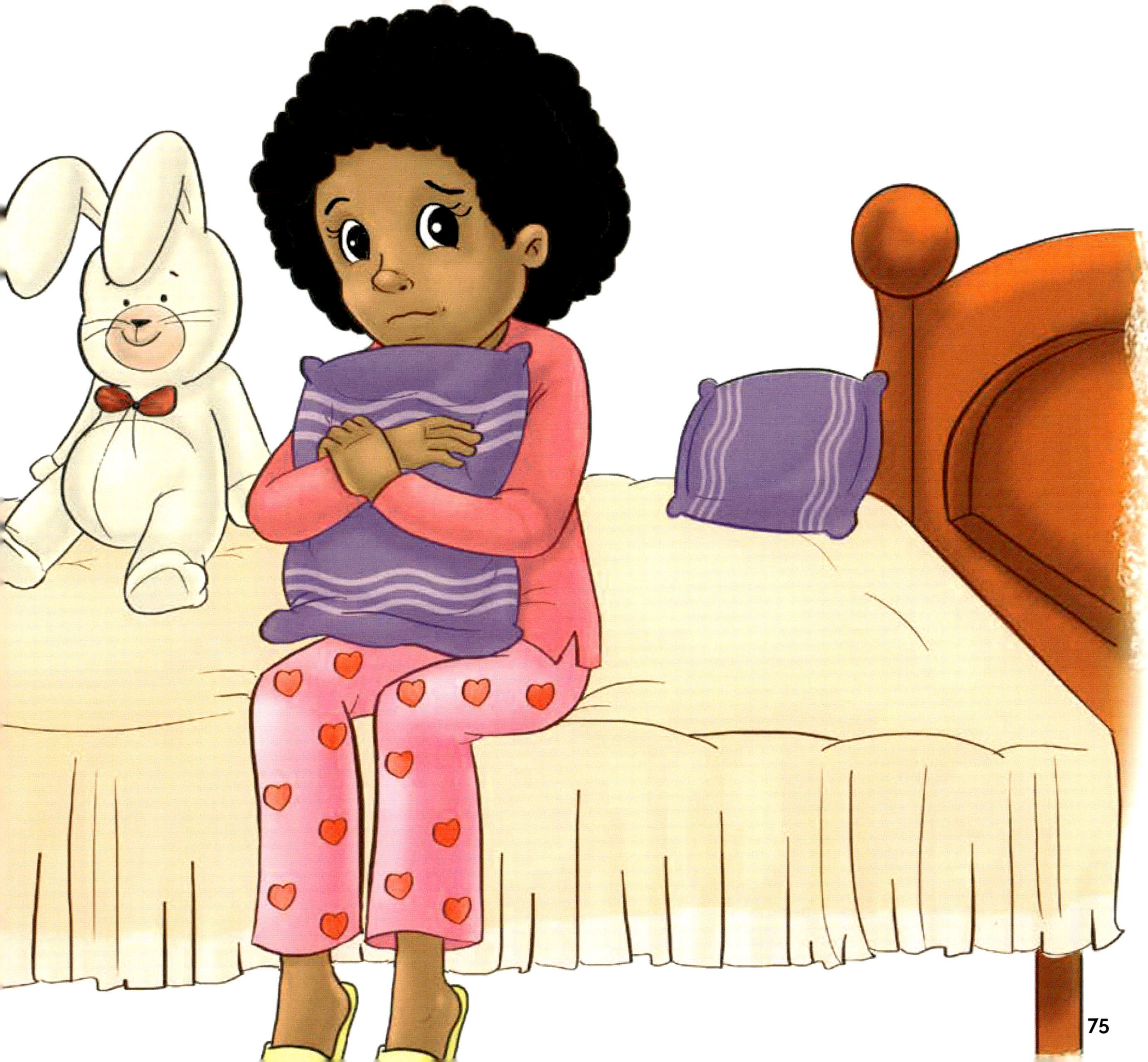

Selma heard and saw three voices, a 2-, 5- and 15-year-old. They came around four years ago. For the first three years, Selma found the voices entertaining and fun to have around.

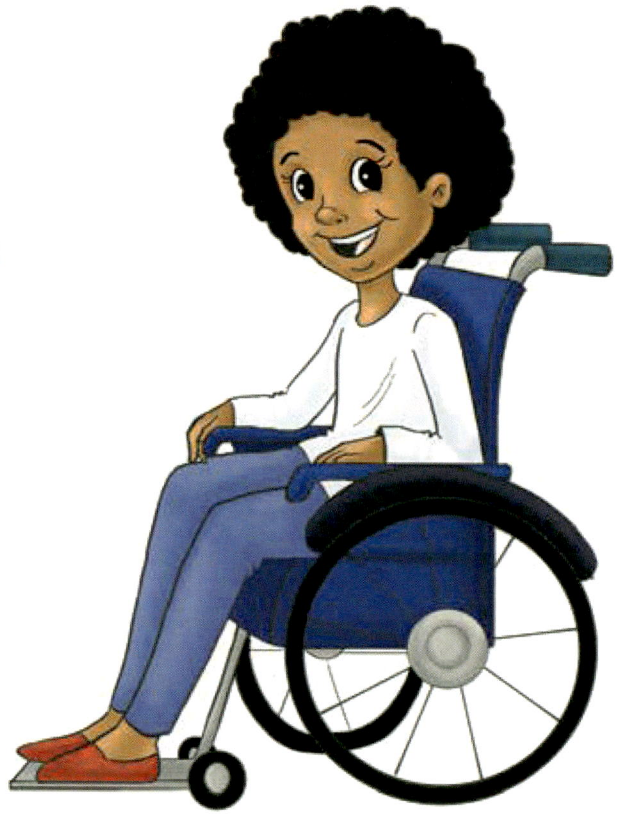

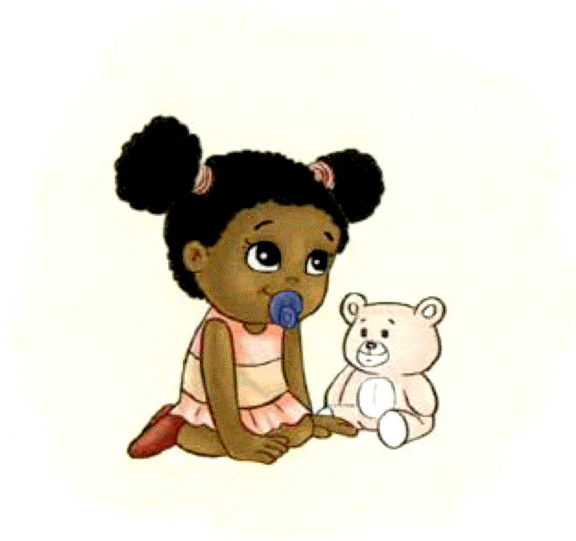

Chuki, the 2-year-old, had a pacifier in her mouth and carried a stuffed teddy bear wherever she went.

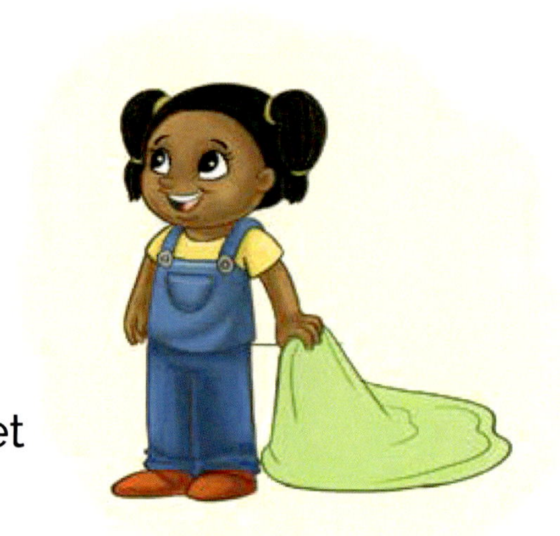

Five-year-old Aisha dragged a blanket around with her all the time

Chuki was the **annoying** complainer who liked to whine like a baby.

Aisha was also **annoying** because of her arguing, screaming and yelling. Chuki and Aisha regularly squabbled and fought over anything and everything.

Often they couldn't resolve their differences and, to make their complaints, they'd run to Jamiyah, the 15-year-old.

Jamiyah tried to reason with them because she truly cared about the kids. No matter how irritating they were, she always kept an eye on the children to ensure their safety.

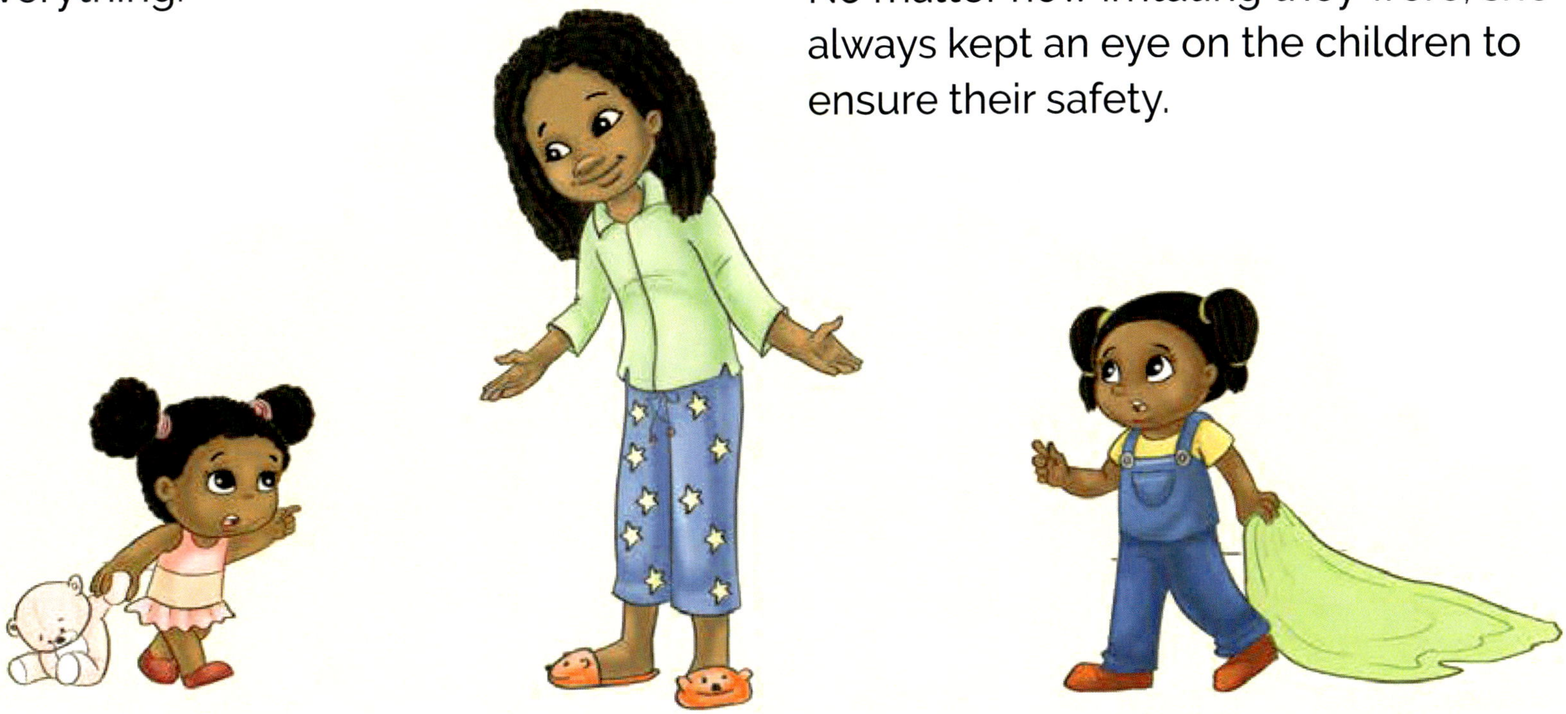

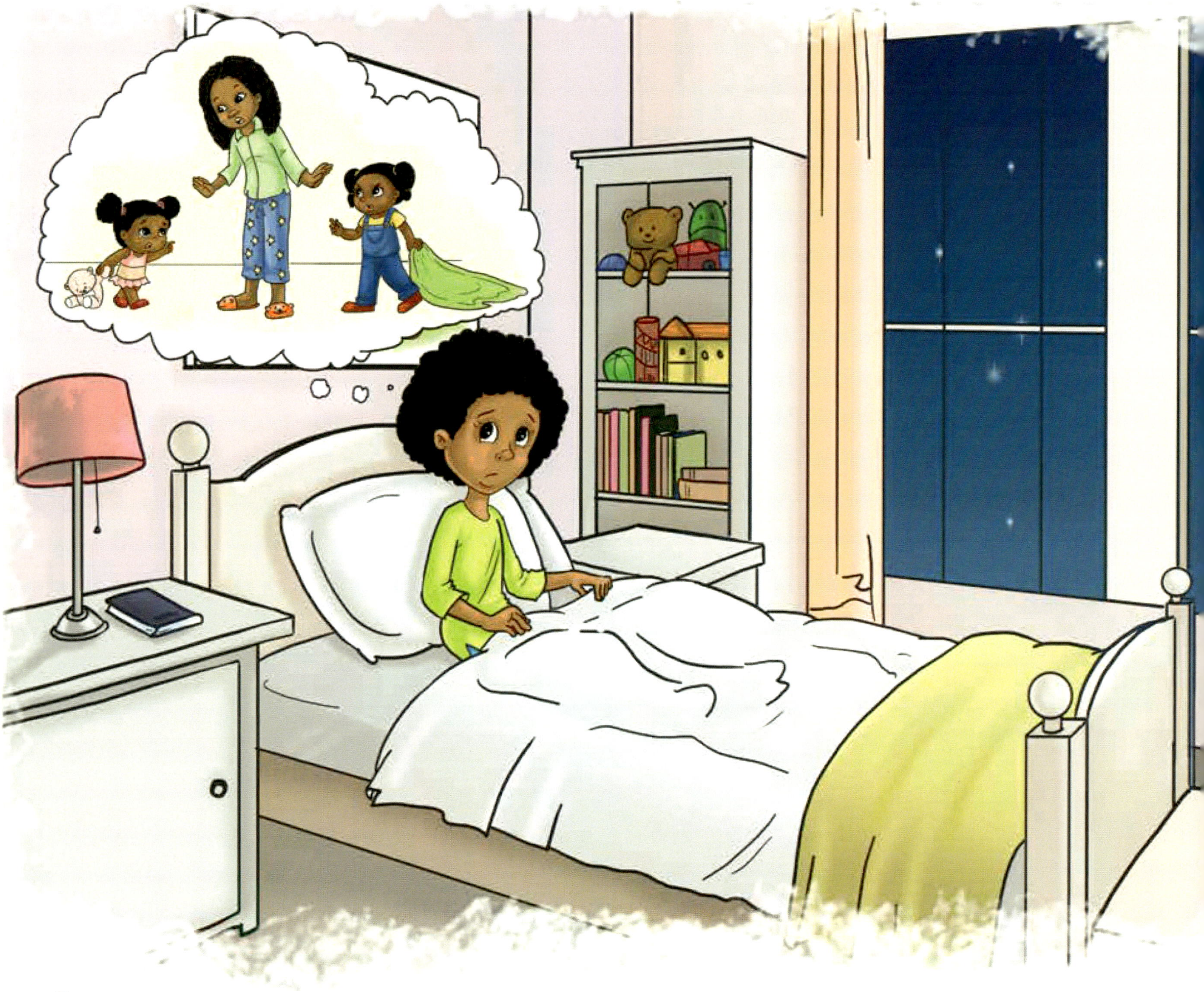

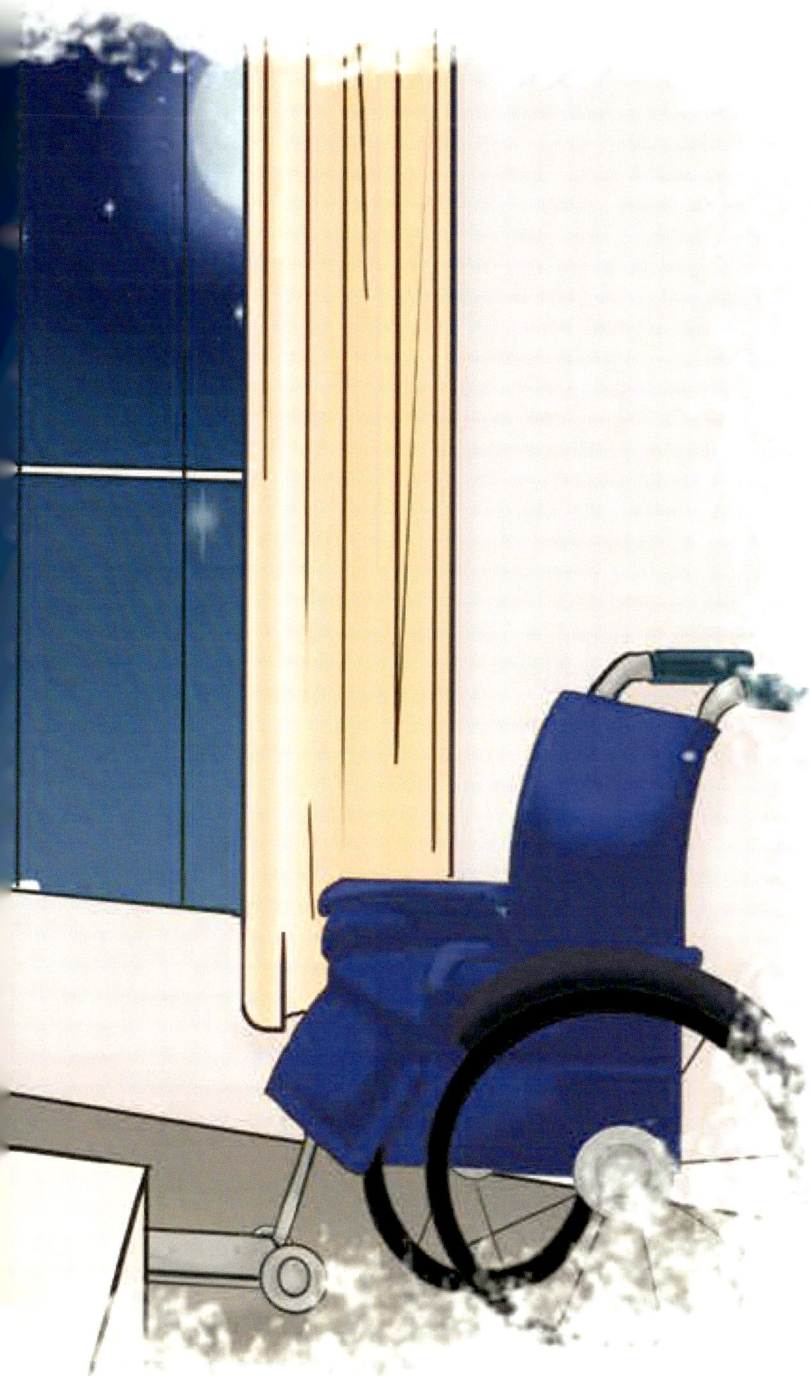

It was during the last year that Selma started having **mixed** feelings about the voices. Sometimes she found them entertaining. Sometimes she found them irritating.

The squabbling, quarreling and jabbering trio entertained Selma when she was bored. But the very squabbling that kept her company when she was alone or in unexciting social situations began to annoy her late into the night.

“I want play pookie-bear,” Chuki would say.

“No, you can't!” Aisha would shout.

Chuki would cry, “You meanie!”

Whiner Chuki and Yeller Aisha would go on and on like this for hours. Jamiyah tried to sort things out between the two, but a lot of the time she could not handle the situation.

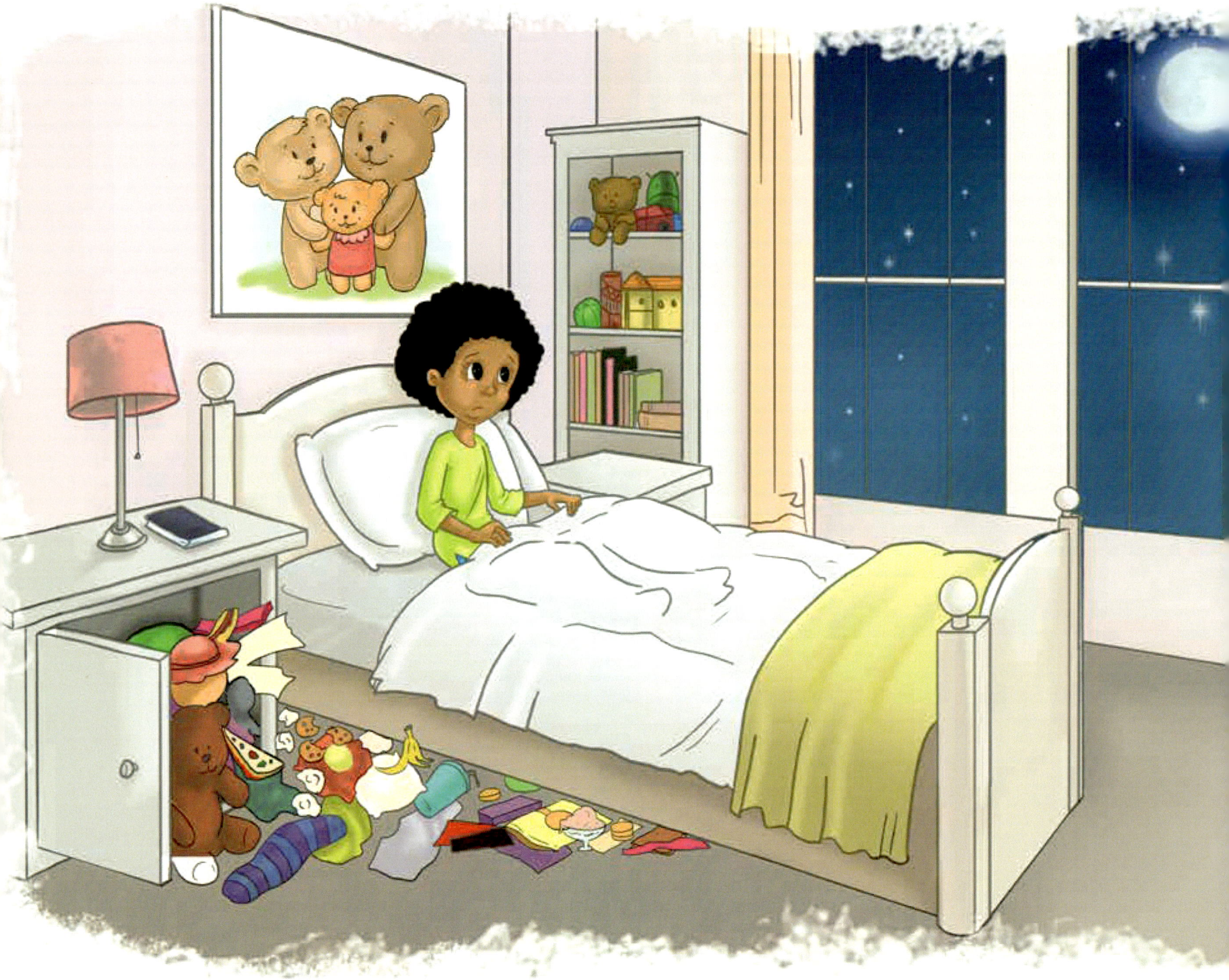

Selma, too, found it hard.

More than once, to solve the problem, Selma went over to the playroom or kitchen and took whatever it was that the yeller and the whiner were arguing over and hid it under the bed or in the closet.

Toy trucks, chocolate bars, squirt guns, cookies, Barbie dolls, ice cream, bananas and bags of chips started piling up in her room.

Besides having to tolerate the squabbling, Selma had a hard time explaining the stashed food, toys and strange smells to her foster mom and dad.

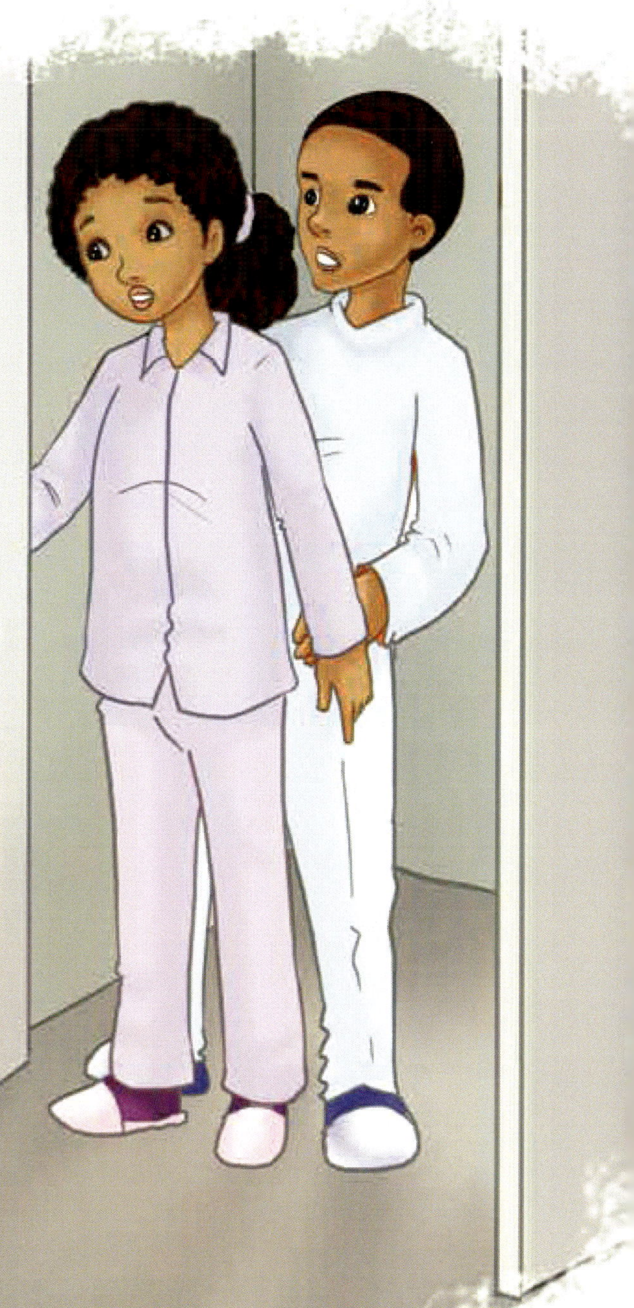

Just before you think Selma, Carlos and I are the only ones who struggled with voices, you should know that Chang heard a voice too.

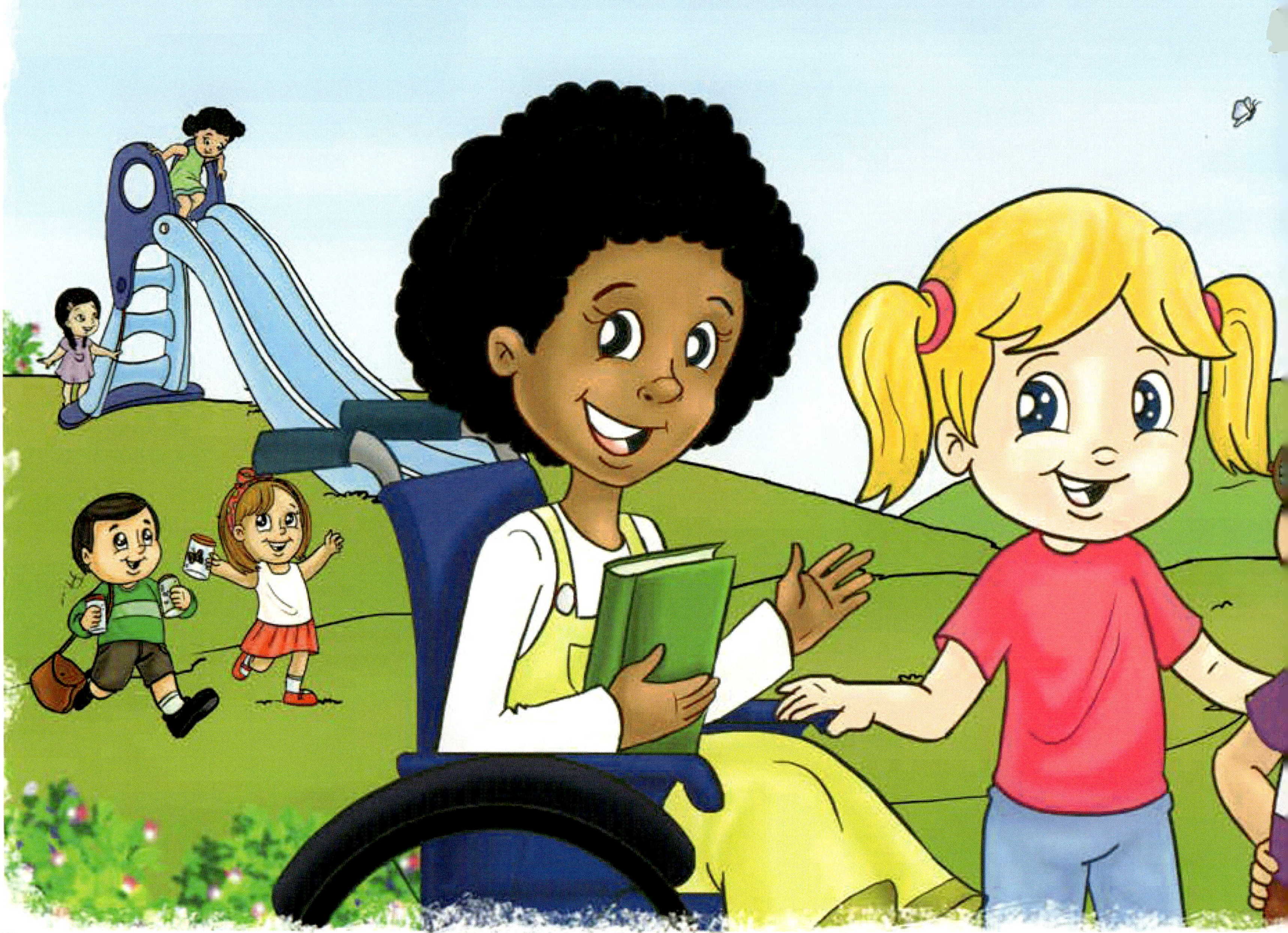

Read on if you would like to hear the story of **Chang's bully.**

If **no, go** on **to Chapter 6.**

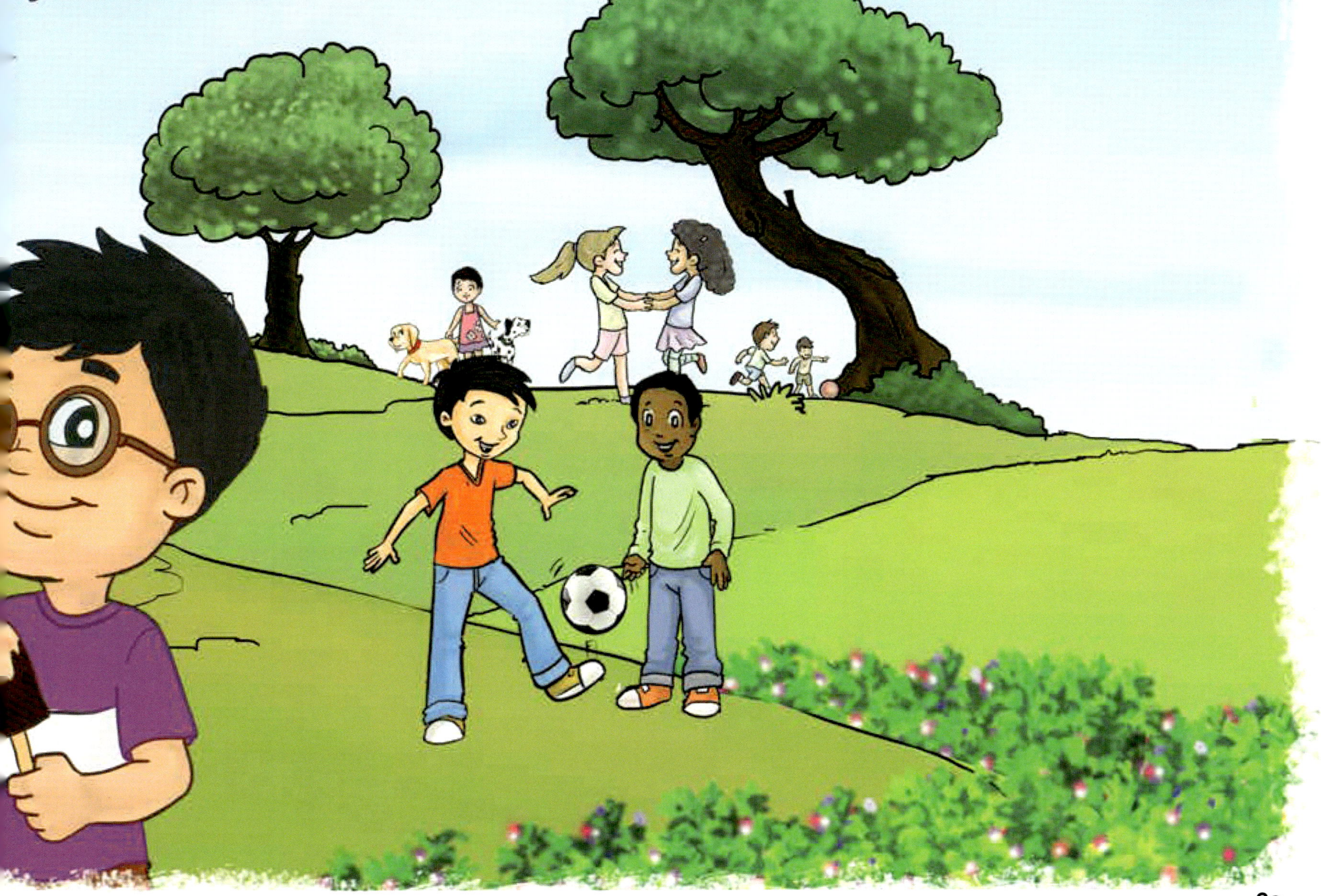

Chapter Four

The Invisible Bully

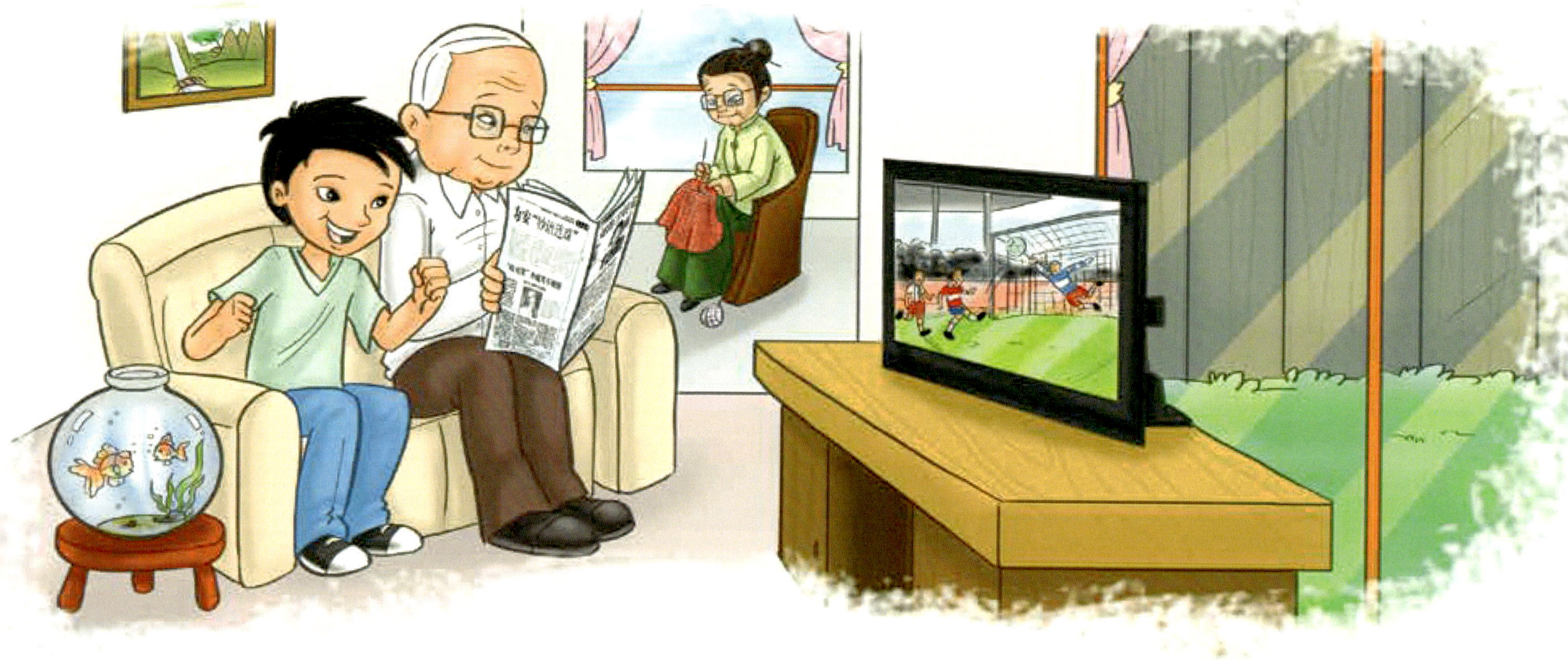

This is Chang Ming Kai. He is 12 years old and lives with his grandparents.

Chang is a huge soccer fan. He watches a lot of soccer on TV and dreams of playing on a team when he grows up. His favorite position is right-back.

He has one other hobby. I bet you won't be able to guess it!

Baking!

Yes, Chang likes to bake! His grandmother lets him bake cookies, cakes and all kinds of sweet stuff.

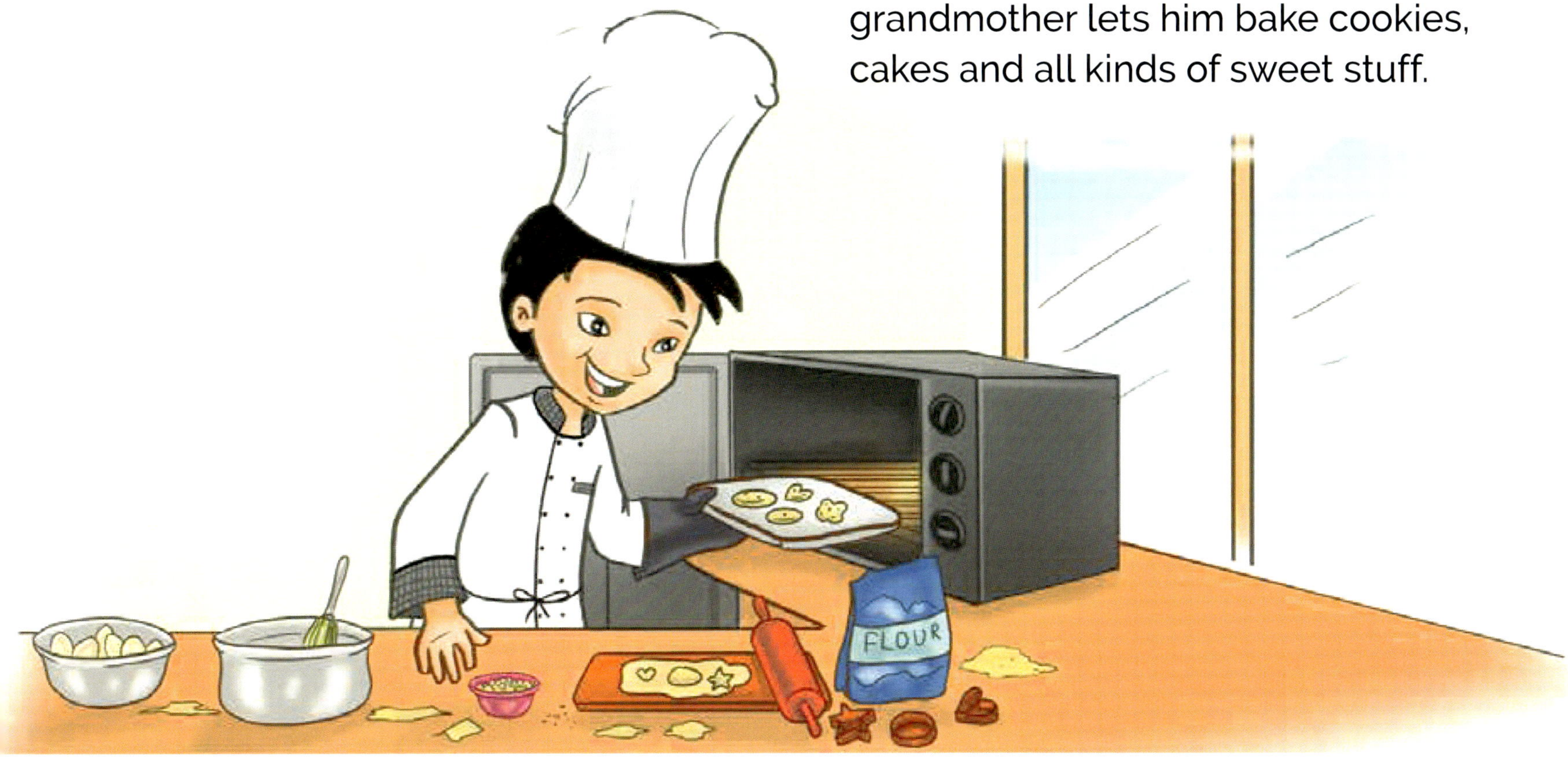

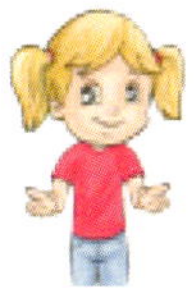

Do you like to do anything that Chang enjoys?
What are your hobbies?

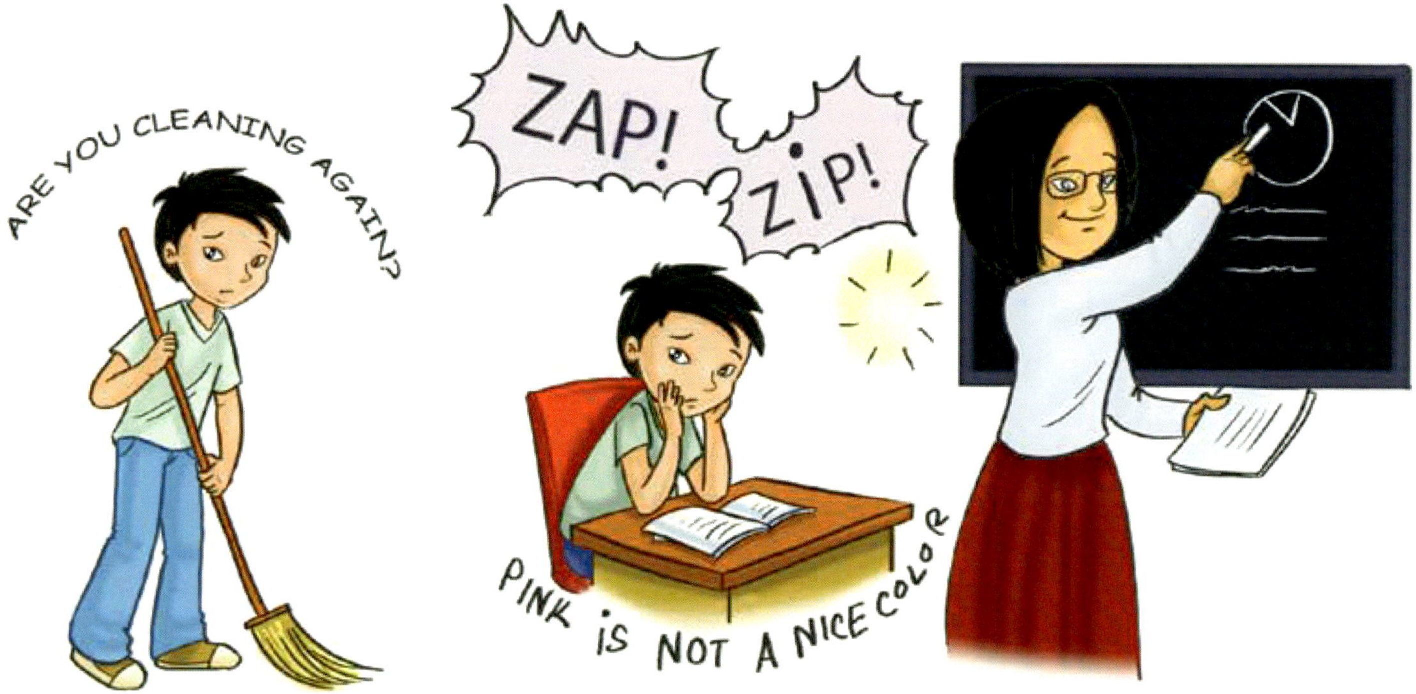

Chang heard a voice too; Mr Charlie Charles.

Mr Charlie showed up whenever, wherever and however he wanted. There was no pattern to his surfacing.

Sometimes he would show up when Chang was doing his chores at home and say things like "Are you cleaning again?"

Sometimes, while Chang was trying to pay attention to his teacher at school, Mr Charlie would make random remarks like "Pink is not a nice color."

While walking to school, Mr Charlie would sing "Twinkle, twinkle, little star..." Chang would feel that in order to drown out Mr Charlie, he had to sing aloud over him.

Sometimes, when watching TV, Chang would hear the sound of a phone ringing, followed by Mr Charlie's voice saying "Hello, hello, hello."

And at other times, he would hear only his name "Chang" being called out.

On top of all of this, Chang also heard bee buzzing noises, sharp and shrill tones, crackling, static and fragmented noises.

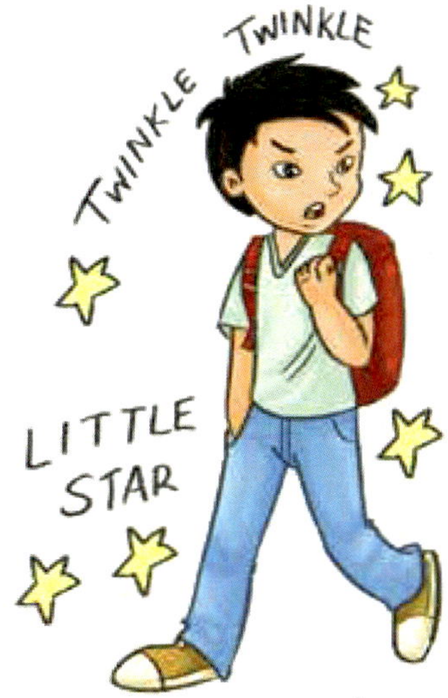

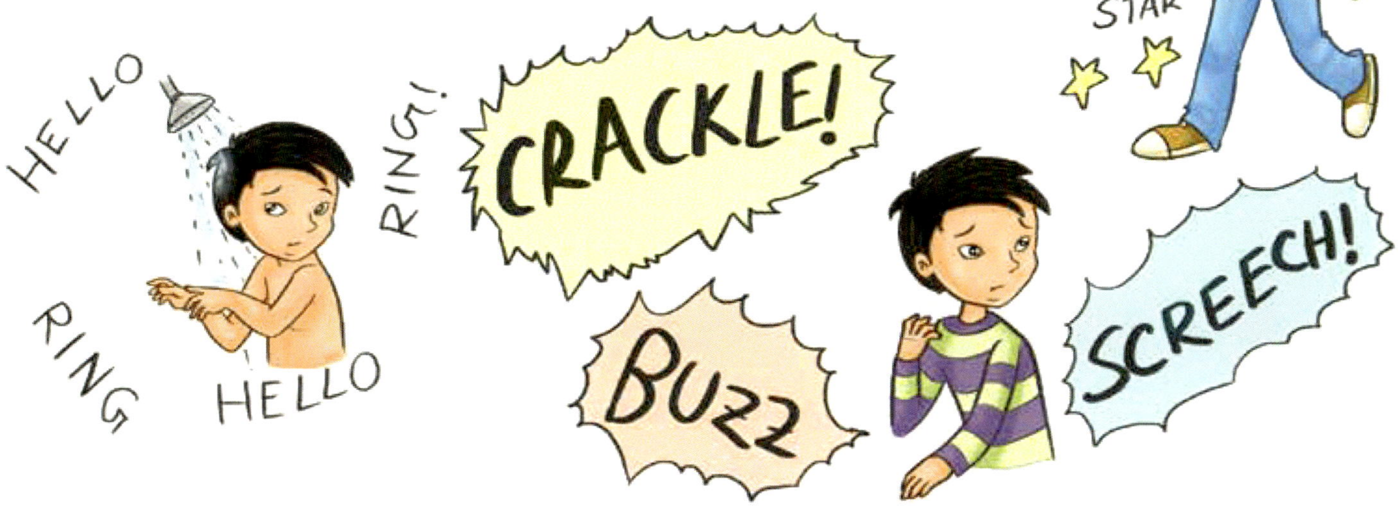

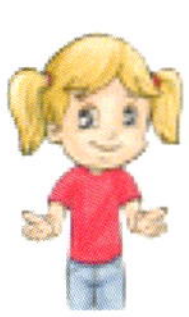

Has this ever happened to you?

What was it like for you?

Unlike Carlos', Selma's and my voice, Chang's voice had no form or figure.

Chang only heard Mr Charlie. He did not see him.

By the sound of Mr Charlie's voice, Chang could tell that he was a grown-up man.

Chang felt **scared** each time the noises and voice showed up. He felt like he was being harassed and bullied by Mr Charlie.

Mr Charlie's noise-making made it hard for Chang to do his schoolwork and house chores.

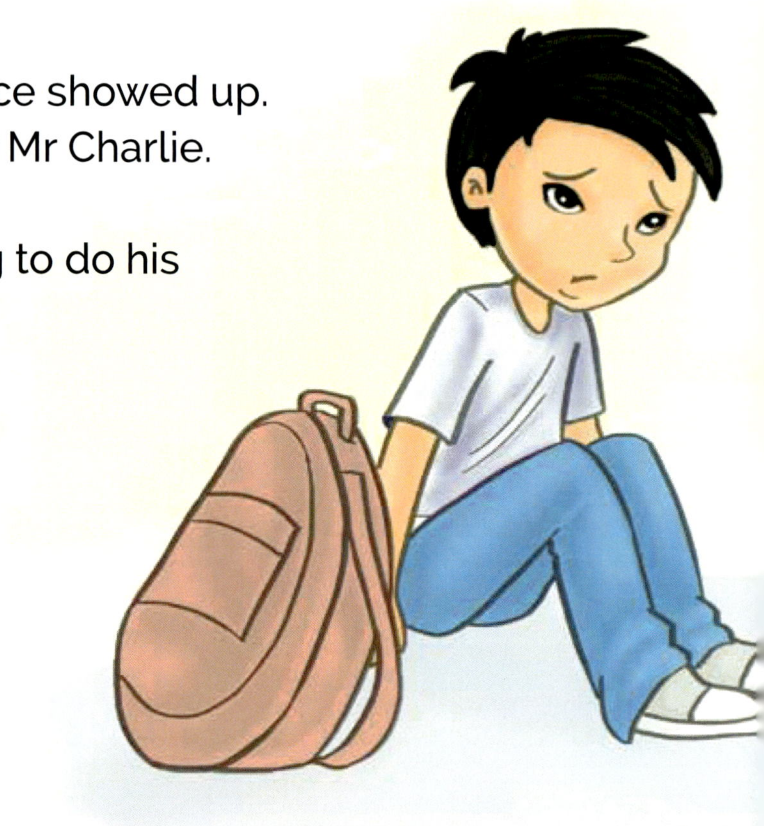

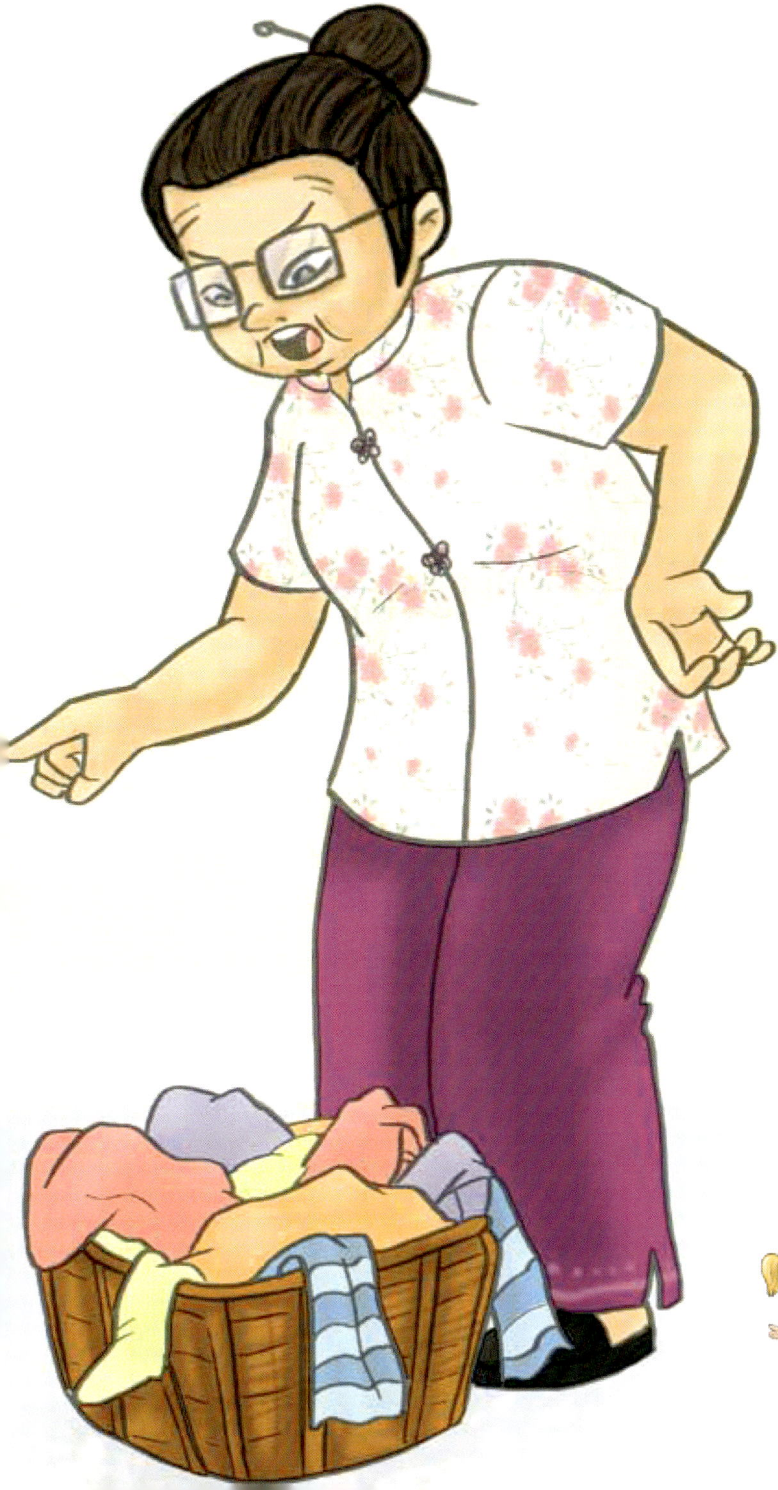

Chang tried hard to avoid hearing Mr Charlie's voice and noises.

Because he worried that Mr Charlie would harass him, he did not take his homework assignments out of his backpack every day.

He would also avoid opening up his exam booklet during class tests, steer clear of watching TV and ignore his grandparents' instructions to do chores.

He was frequently found just staring at "nothing."

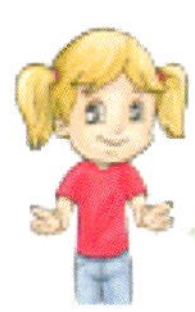

Does your voice interrupt your tasks?
Does it get in the way of things in your life?

Chang's behaviors disappointed his teachers and grandparents.

They thought that he was just using Mr Charlie as an excuse to get out of doing what he needed to.

They didn't believe that Mr Charlie existed in Chang's life.

Chang slowly stopped telling his grandparents and teachers about Mr Charlie's intrusive noises.

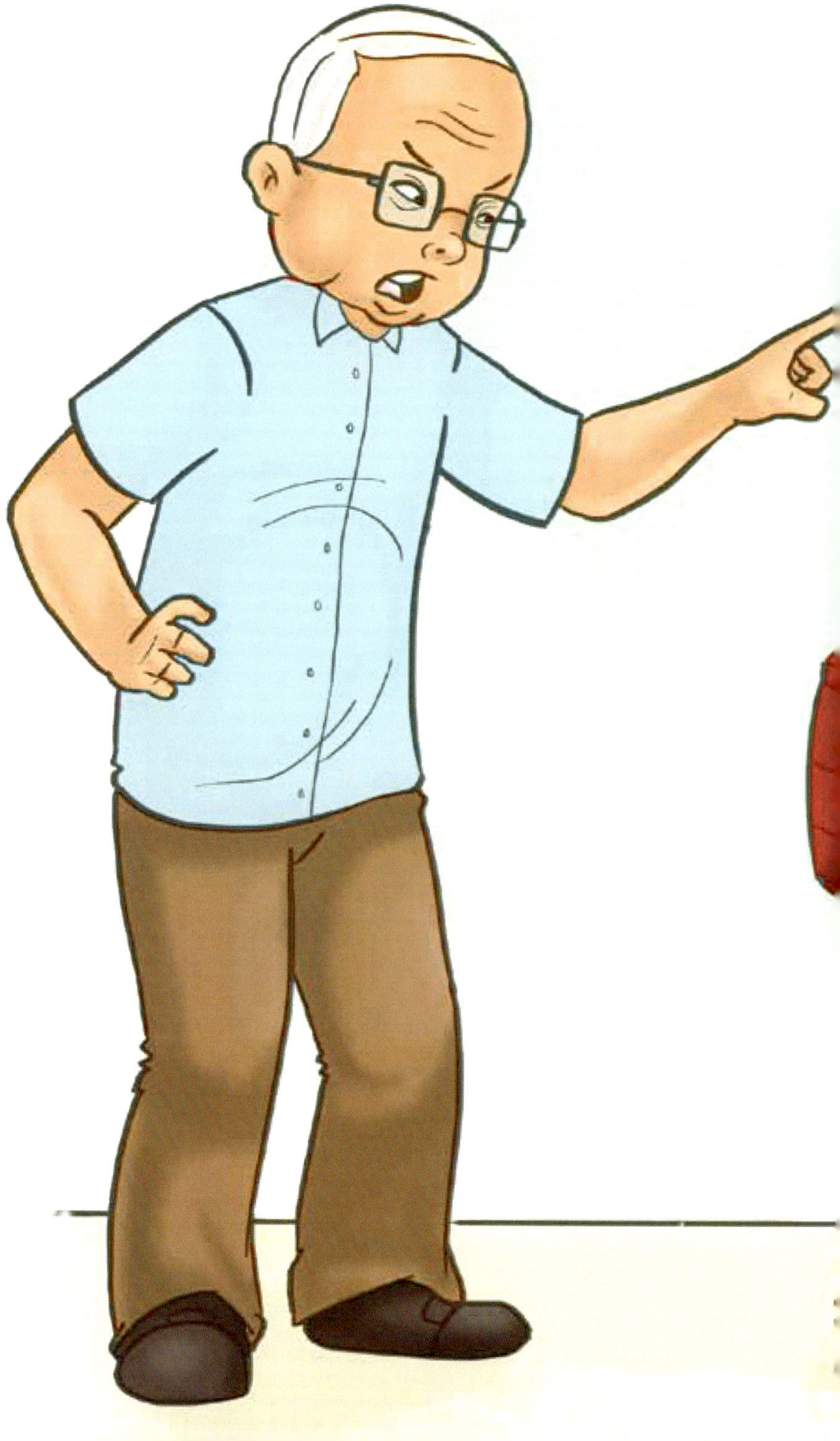

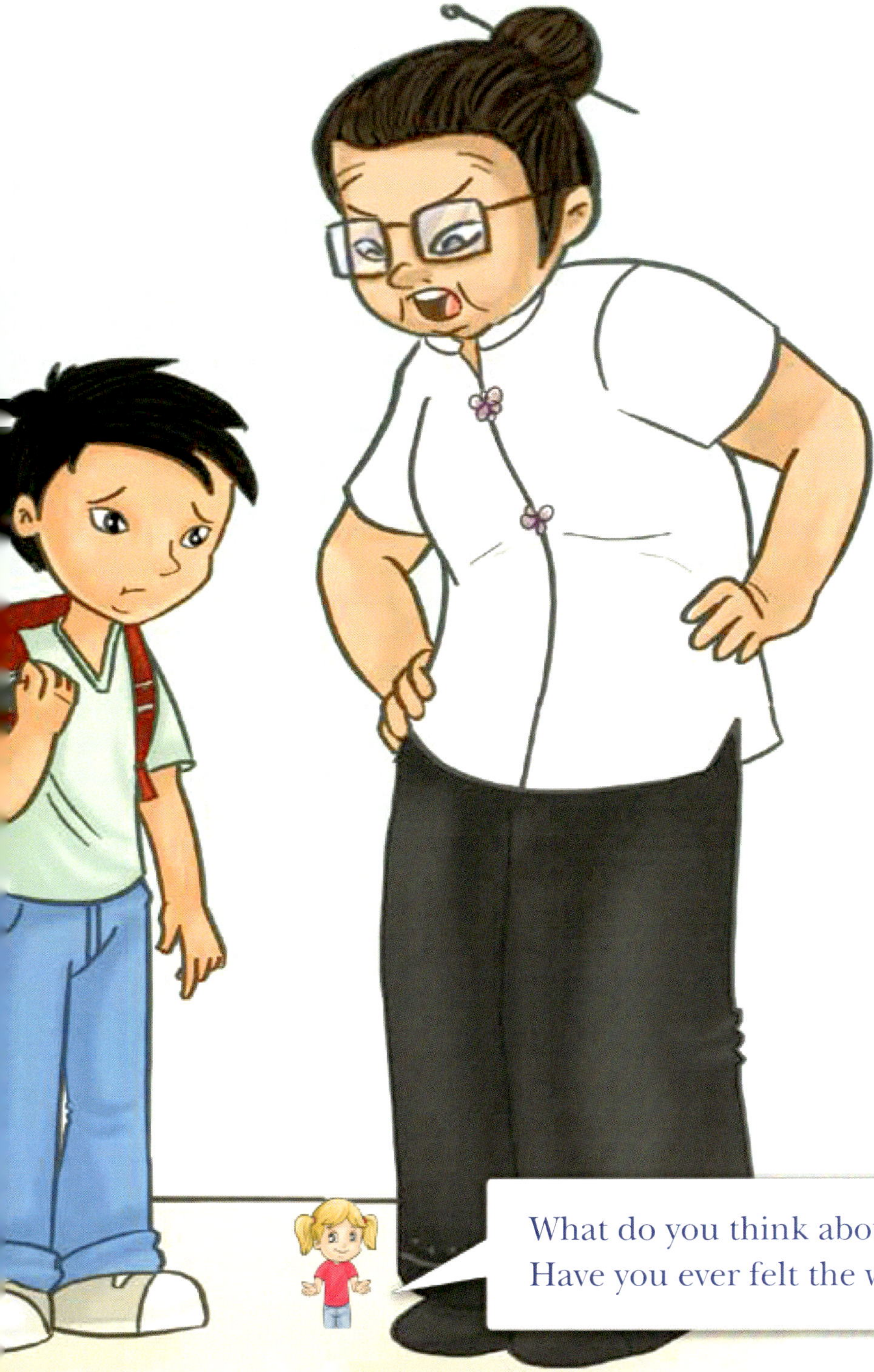

Many many times Chang wished that Mr Charlie would just disappear into thin air.

But he did not know how to make that happen.

He felt so **angry** at himself and Mr Charlie.

Chang tried to tell himself to forget Mr Charlie. But that, too, didn't work!

What do you think about Chang's situation?
Have you ever felt the way Chang did?

One day, Chang made a discovery.

Each time he ate something, the voice vanished for a while. So he began to eat frequently.

Sometime later, Chang's doctor told his grandmother that Chang was becoming too big because he was eating too much.

Chang needed to go on a diet to manage his weight.

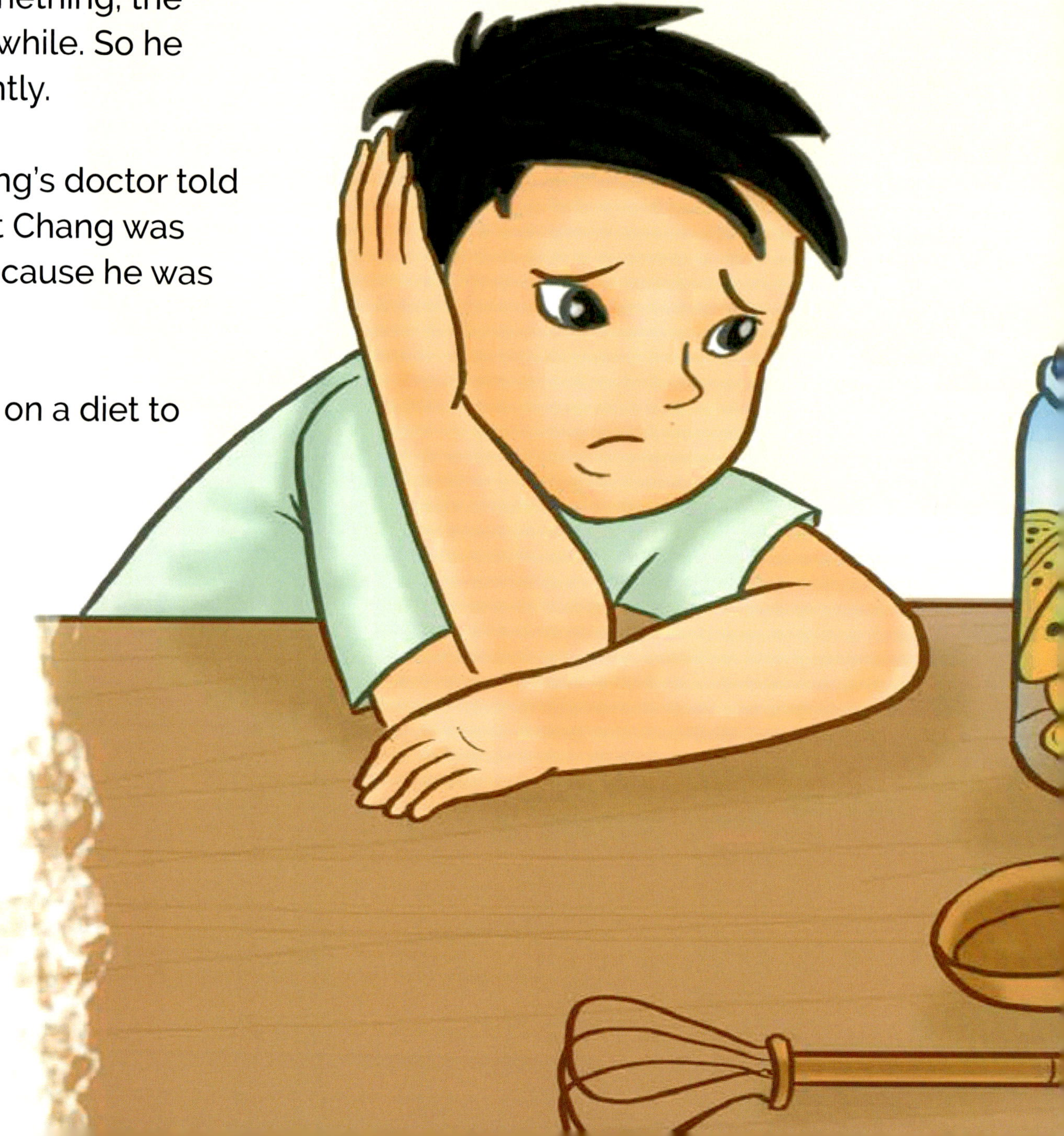

With the food restrictions, Chang could not eat or bake what he wanted or when he wanted.

He did not feel that he was in charge of his own life or his voice.

He started wondering if he was worth anything.

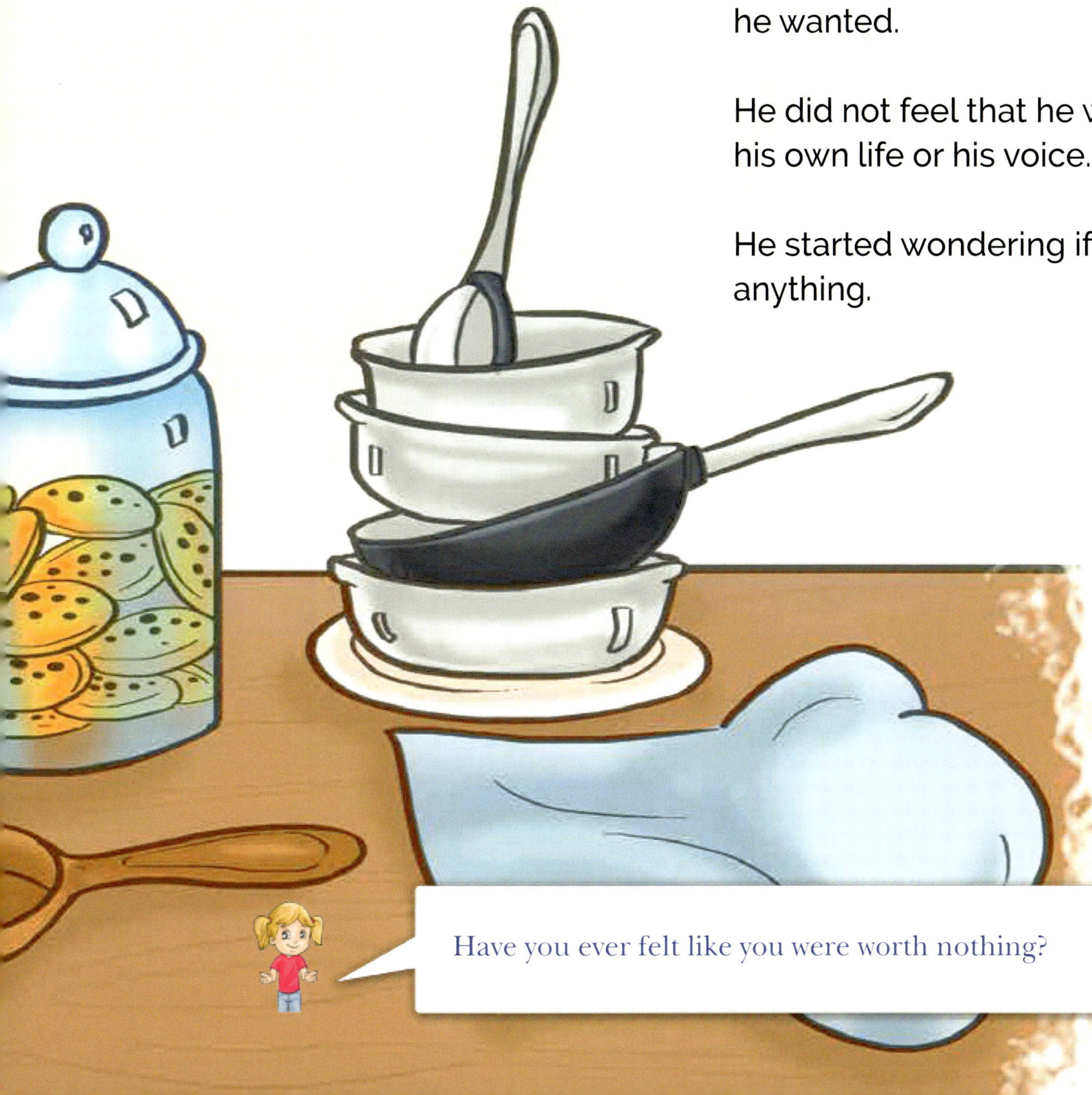

Have you ever felt like you were worth nothing?

So, you see, you're not the only one.

Would you like to hear one last story of a sweet but sad little girl who also heard a voice?

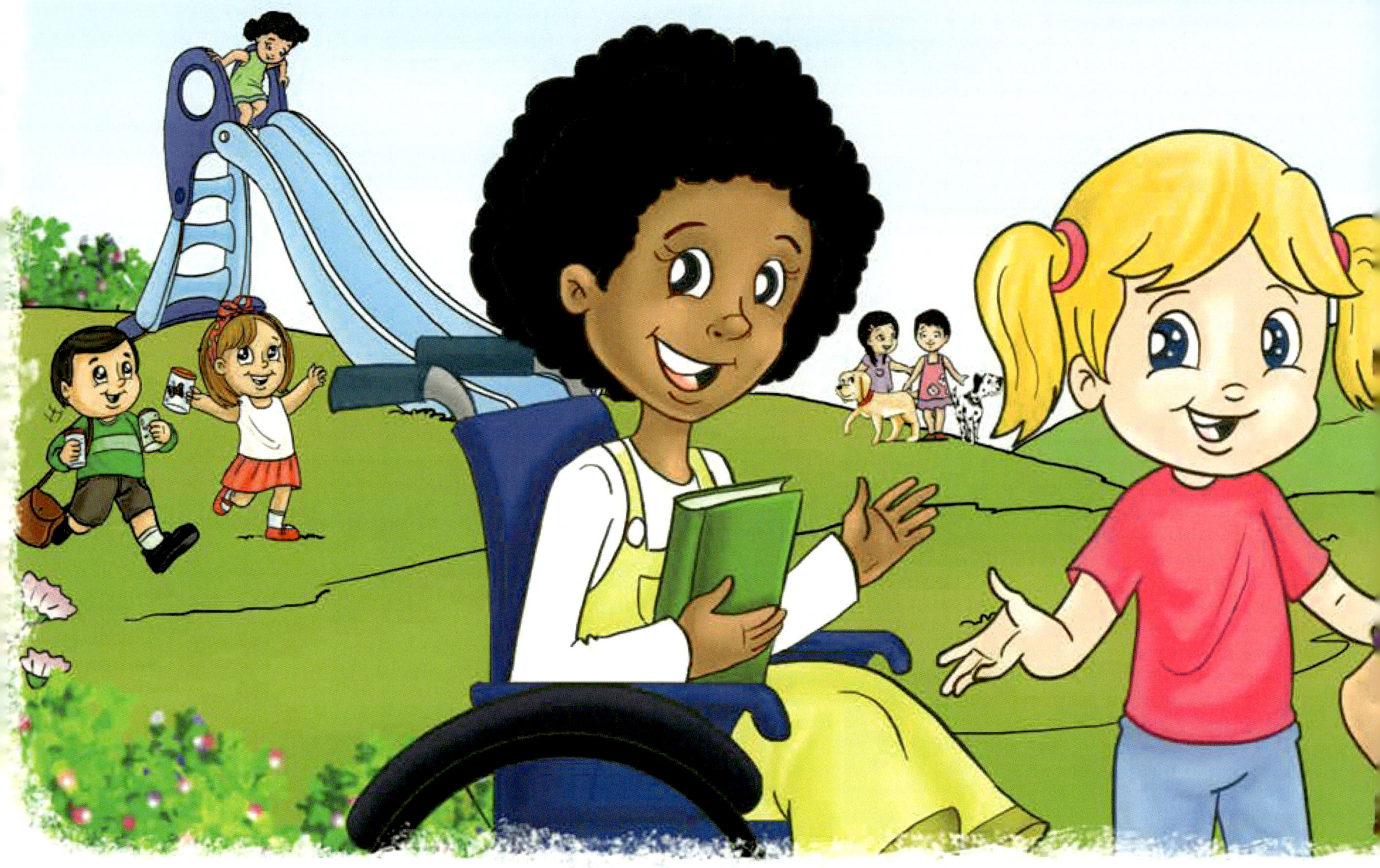

If **yes, read on.**

If **no, skip to Chapter 6.**

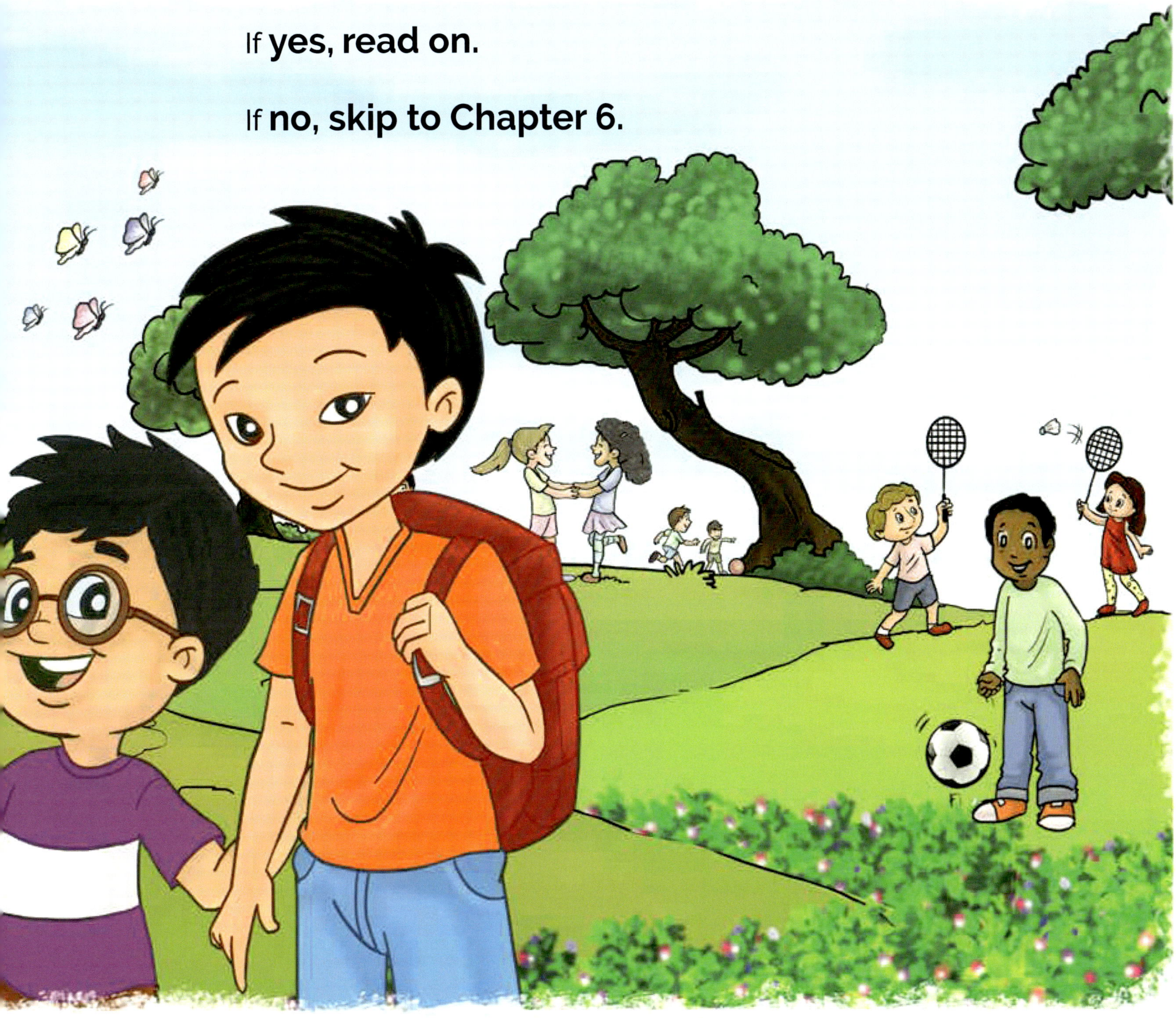

Chapter Five

I Miss You Mommy

Her real name is Leila but her father's nickname for her is La-la.

La-la is 4 years old.

Six months ago, her mother died quite suddenly. She now lives alone with her father.

La-la likes playing house and dress-up. She also likes it when someone reads books to her.

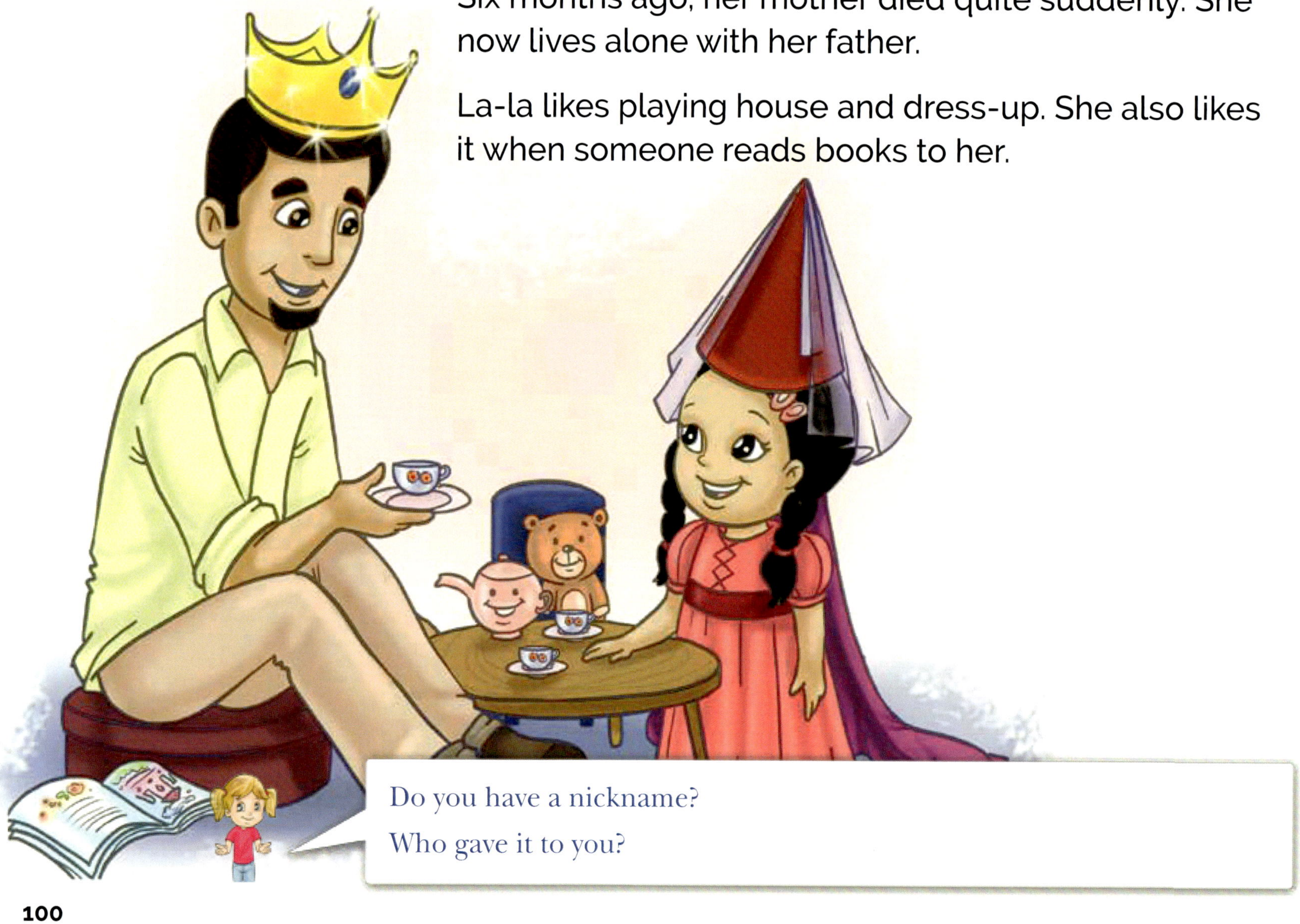

Like Carlos, Selma, Chang and I, La-la heard a voice too.

Soon after her mother's passing, La-la started seeing her mom's figure and hearing her voice, especially at bedtime.

The voice told La-la that she missed her. "I love you, my dear. You're the best daughter a mother could ever have."

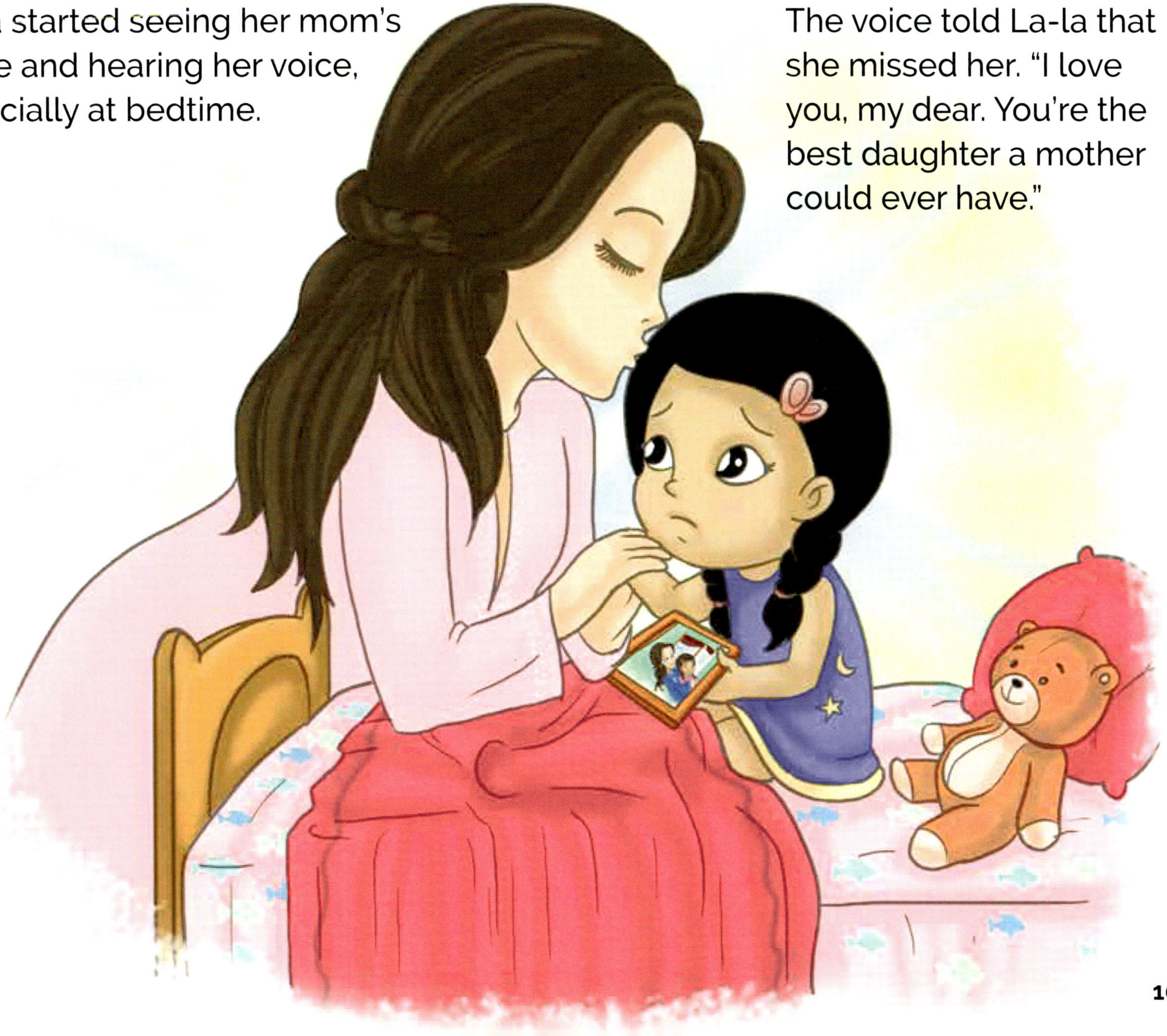

La-la sometimes felt her mom stroking her hair and heard her say that she worries about her not eating well.

From time to time, La-la even talked back to the voice.

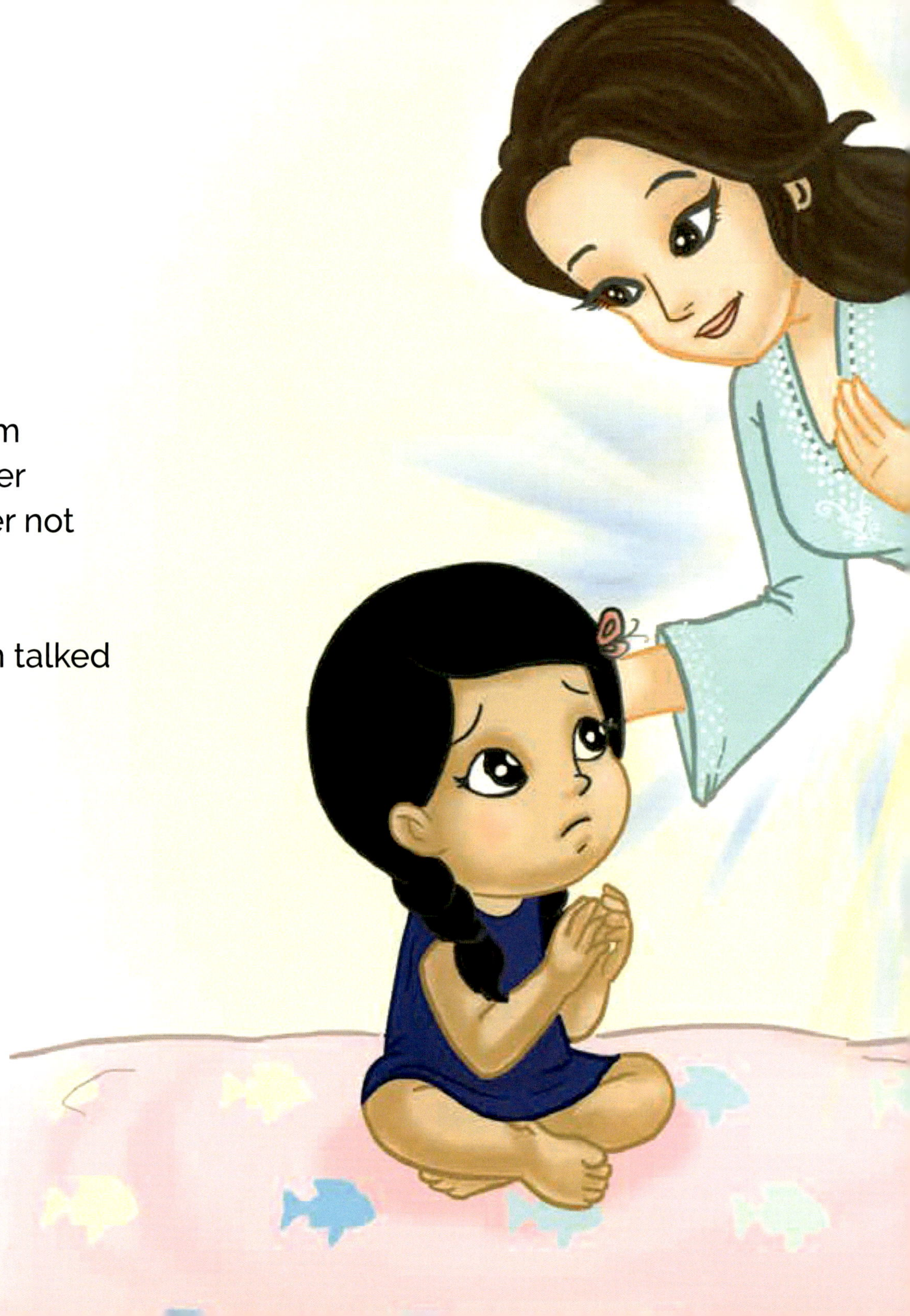

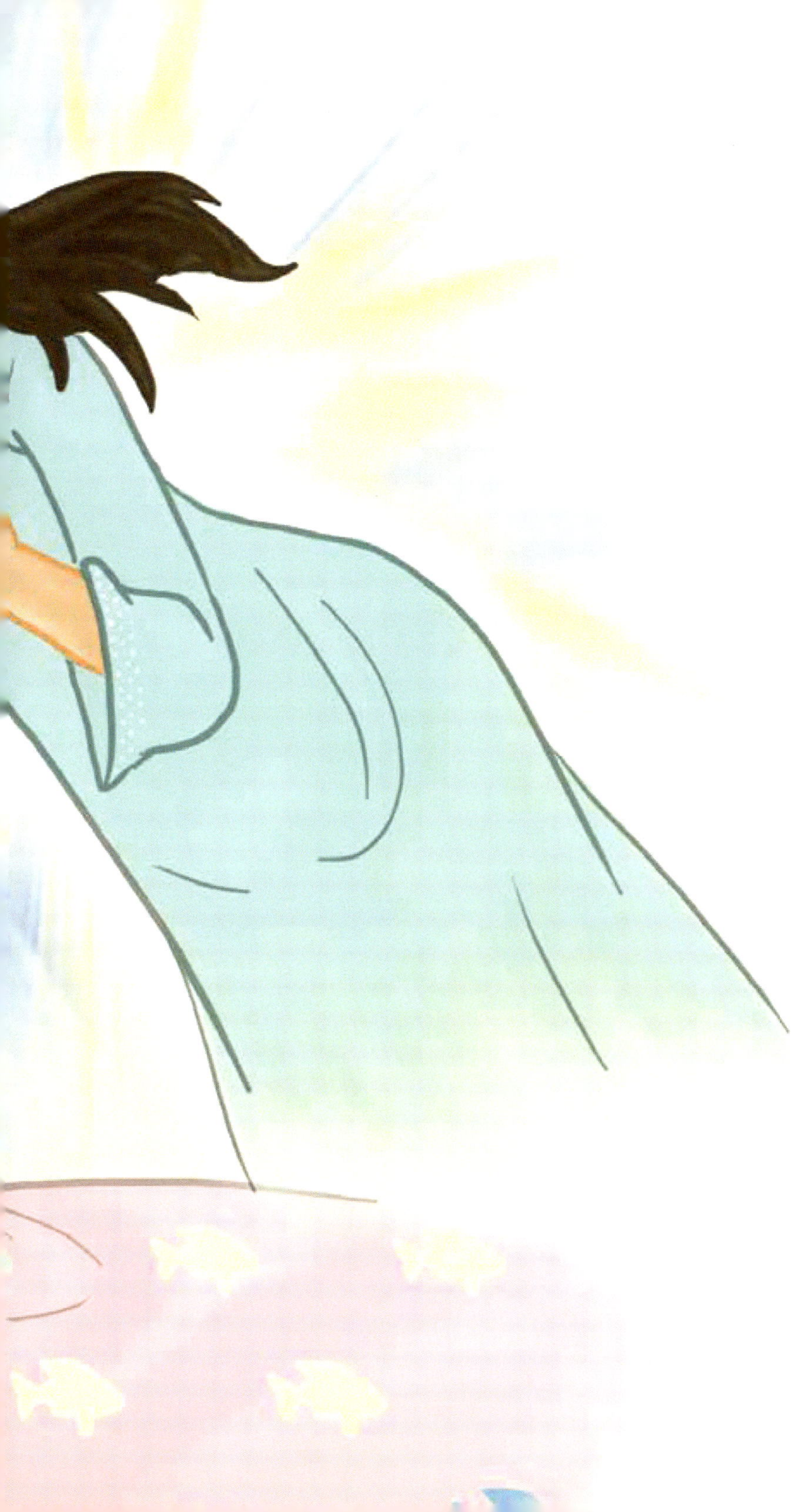

She really liked the voice. She looked forward to bedtime every night.

“I’m sorry for all the bad things I did. I miss you so very much, Mommy. Please, please Mommy, come back. I promise to be good forever,” she’d say.

A few times, La-la's father heard her talking out loud. He went into her bedroom and was surprised!

There was no one there besides La-la!

When he asked La-la who she was talking to, she shrugged her shoulders and said, "No one."

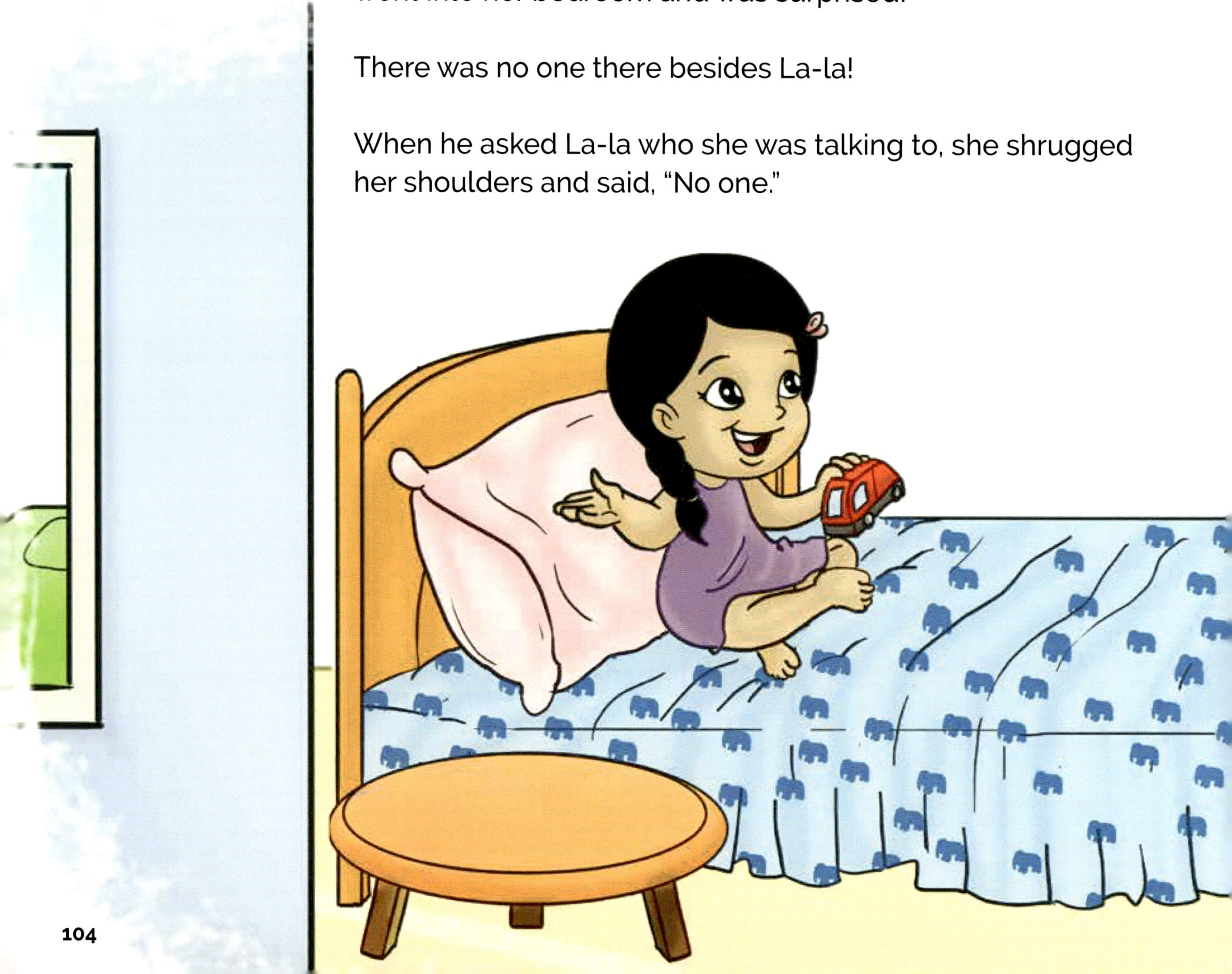

Although La-la found it hard to fall asleep and get a good night's rest when she heard her mother's voice, she found the voice comforting.

But she never told her father about it because she thought he would disapprove.

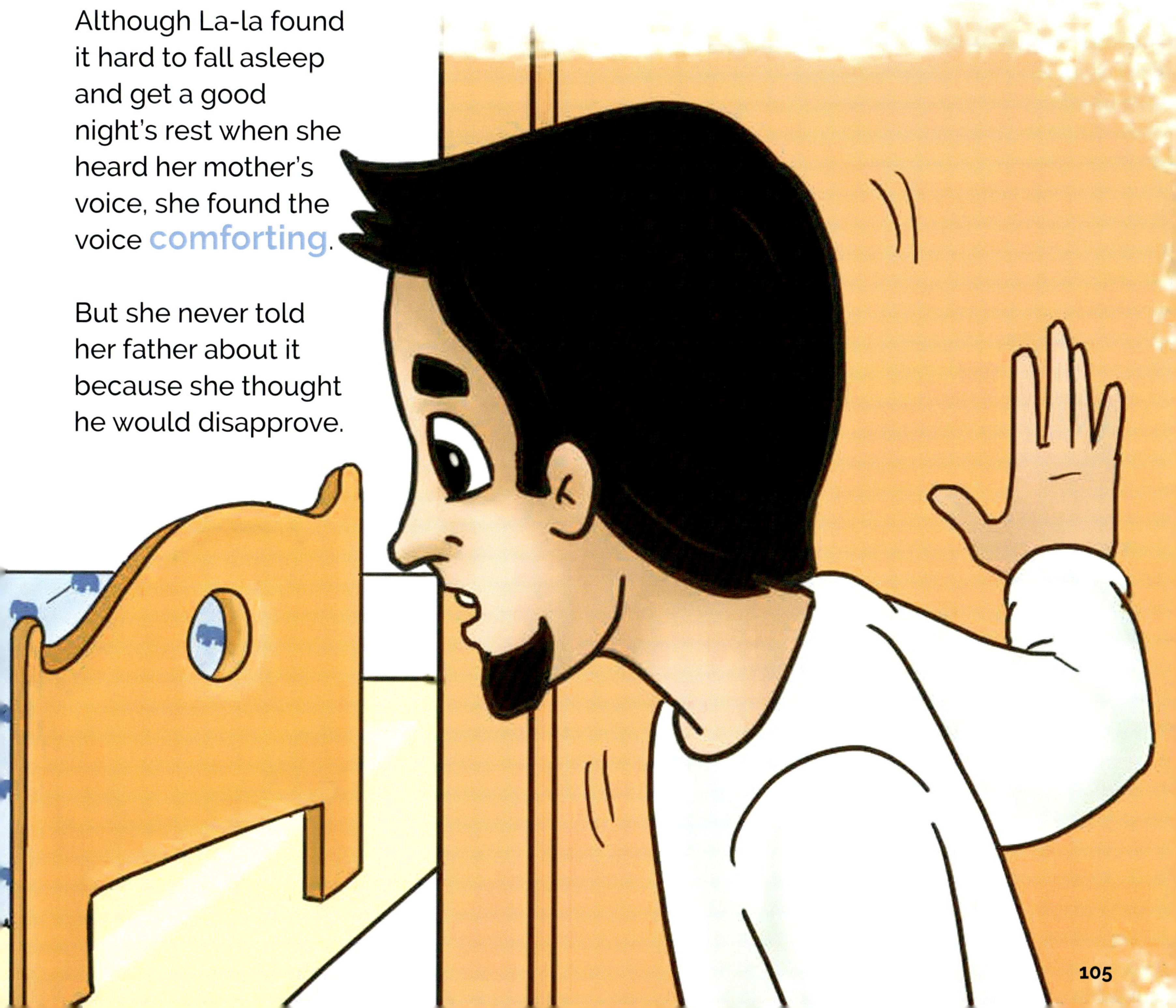

Her father became really worried after the third time he heard La-la talking to "no one."

Finally, he took La-la to see a counselor for help.

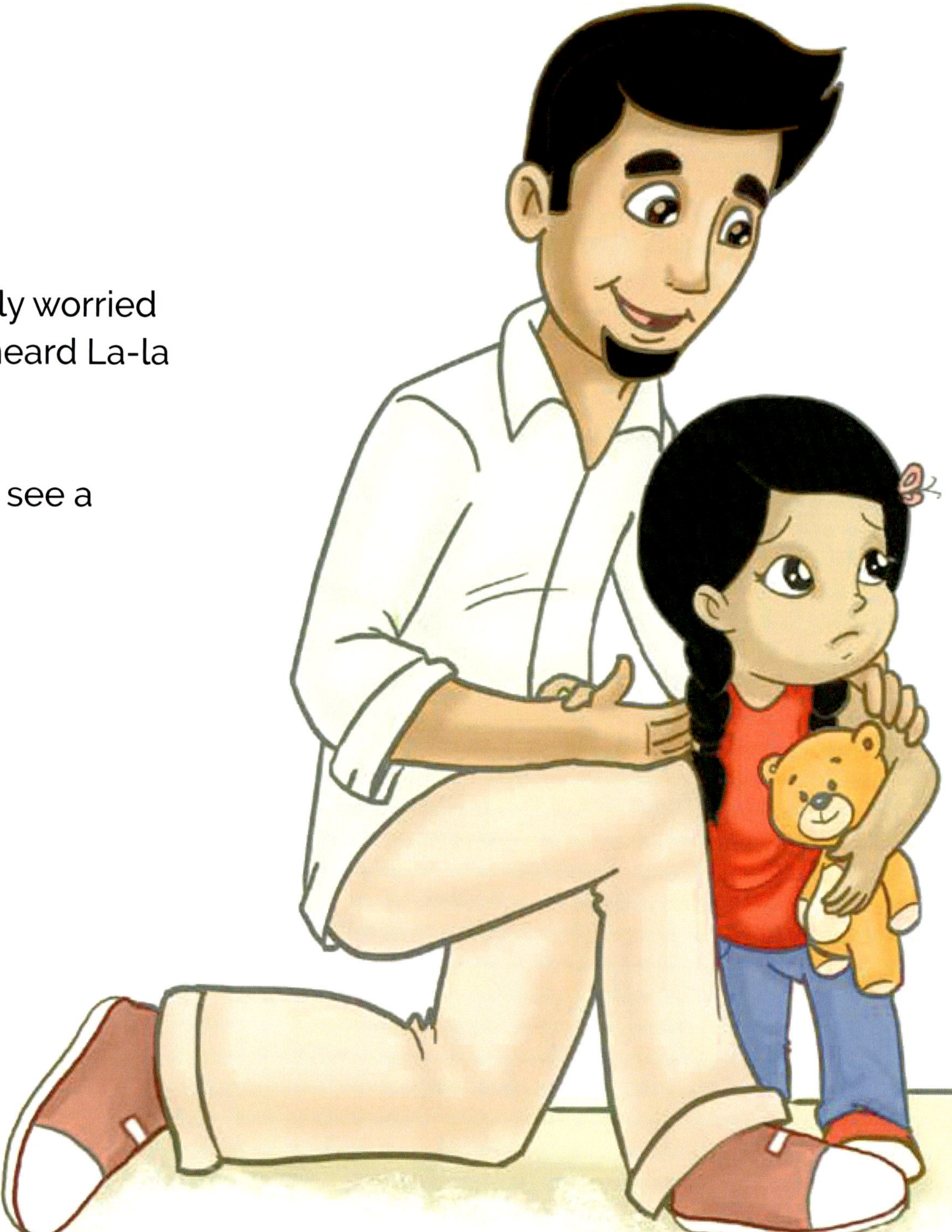

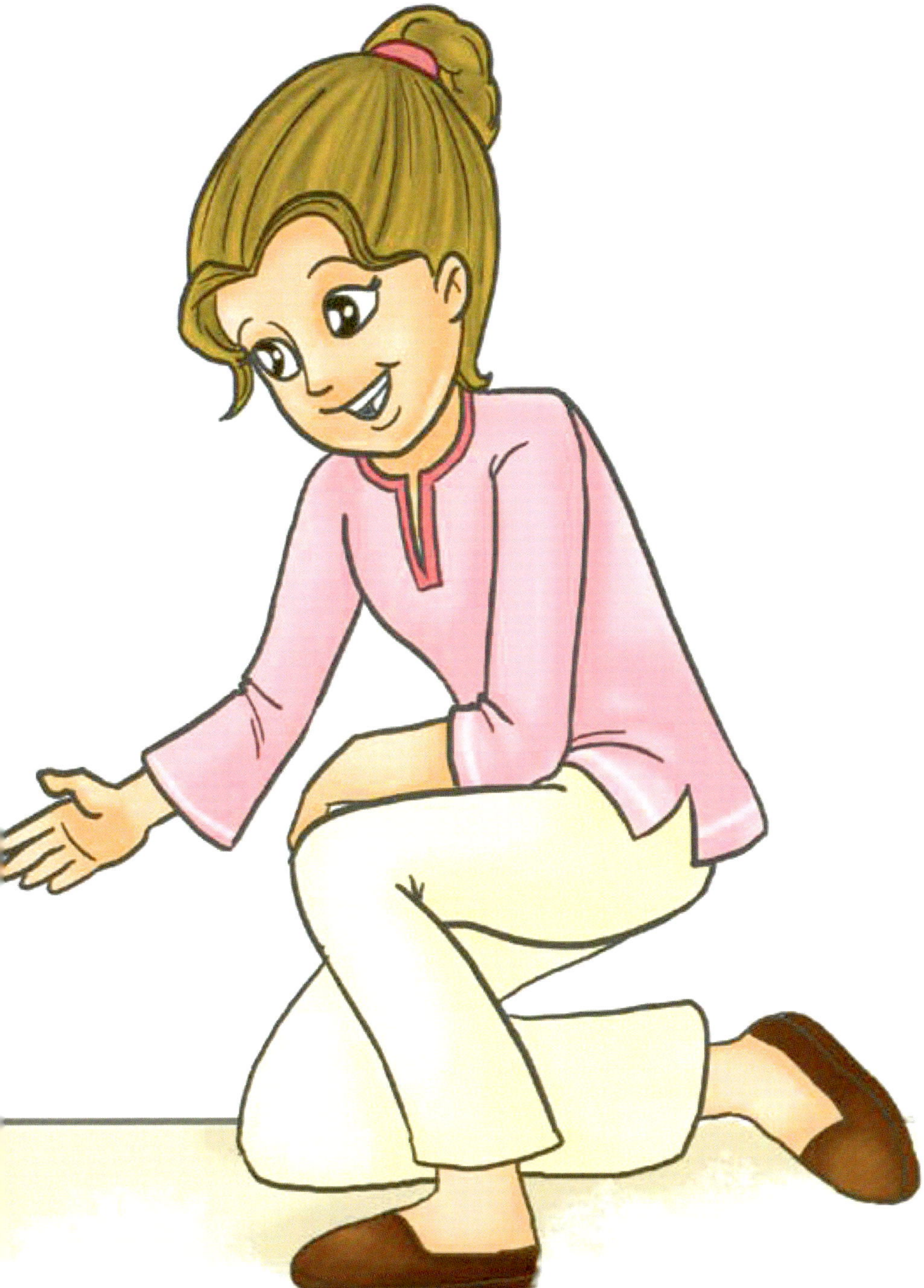

Now that you have heard about different sorts of voice hearing from different kids, I hope you see that you're not the only one.

You're not alone, that's for sure!

All kinds of kids hear voices.

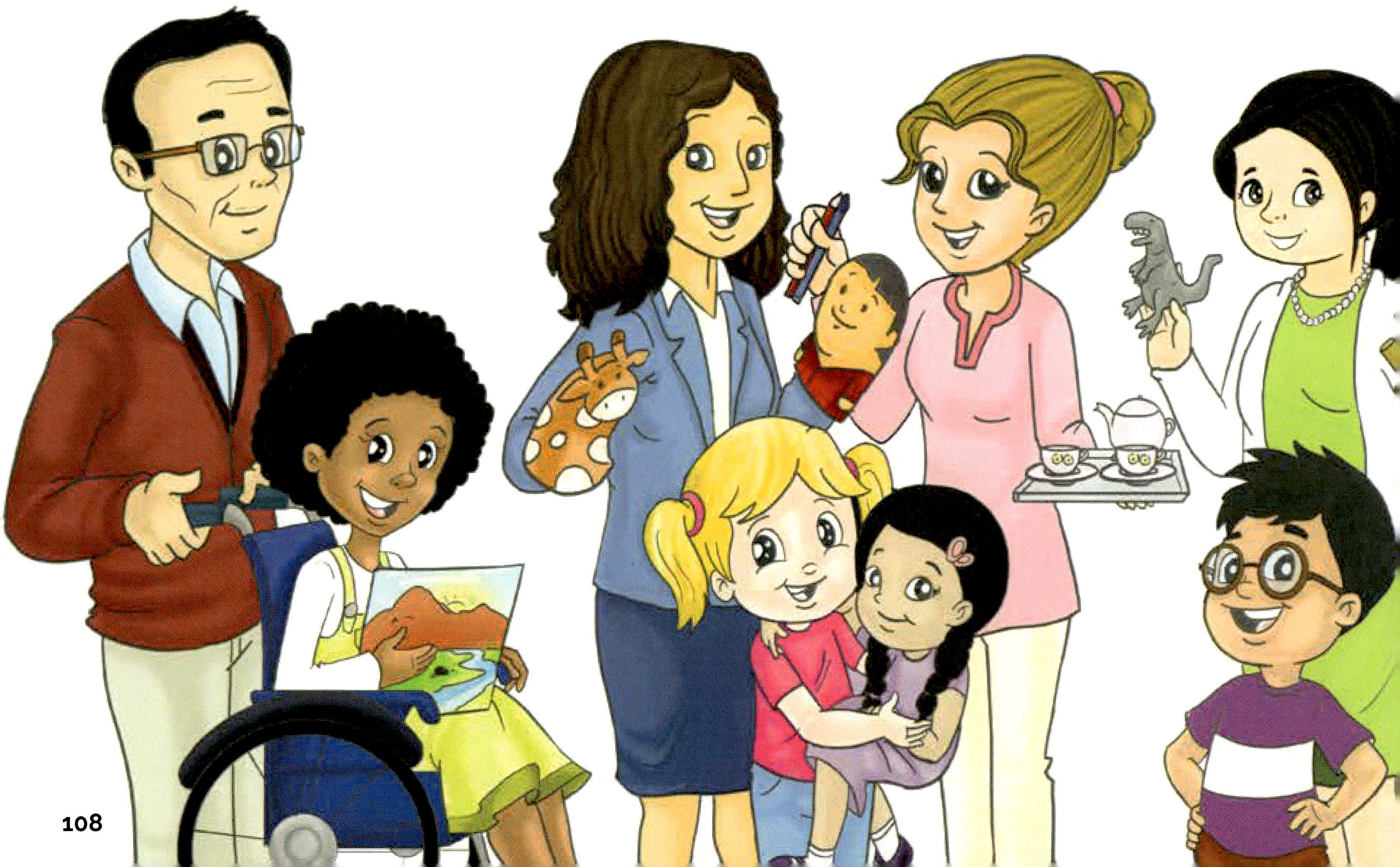

Carlos, Selma, Chang, La-la and I hear voices too!

We're not weird! And you're not weird either!

We're all special!

And you know what? Mr Jones, my favorite teacher, was right.

Counselors can help in these types of situations.

Thanks to his suggestion, my parents and I went to see Amy and learned all about voices and managing them.

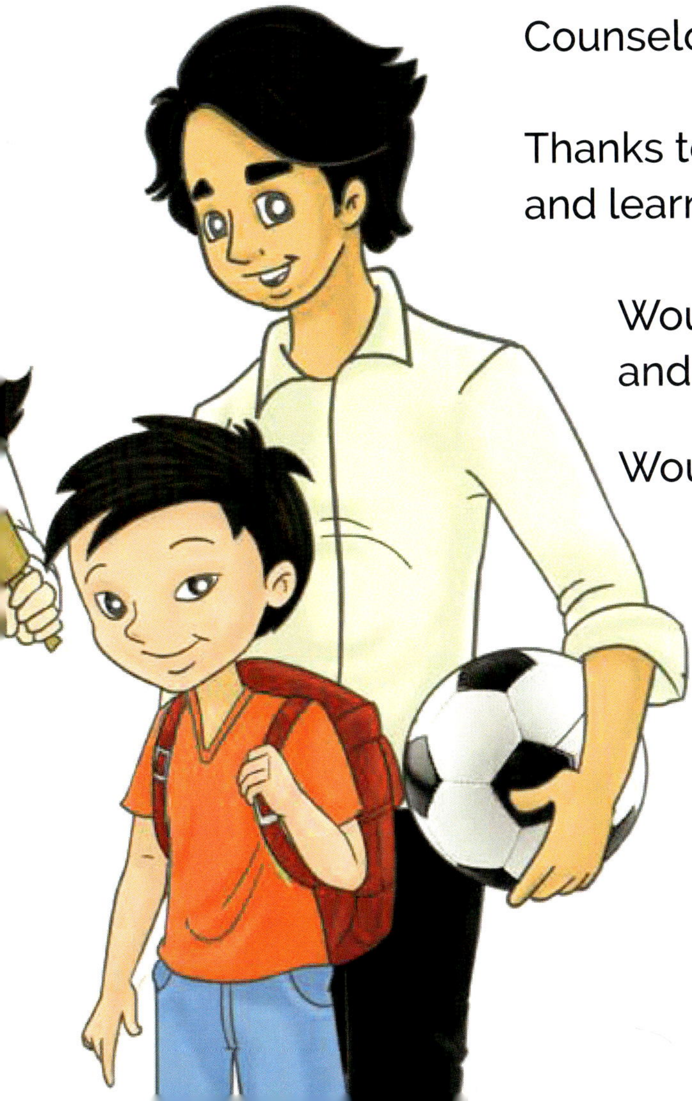

Would you like to know how Carlos, Selma, Chang, La-la and I dealt with our voices?

Would you like to know how to manage your voices?

If **yes, read on.**

Chapter Six

Managing Voices

Hi! Welcome back!

Just in case you have forgotten my name, it's Susie!

Carlos, Selma, Chang, La-la and I realized it was such a relief to talk about the voices and share our experiences with someone we trusted, like our counselors.

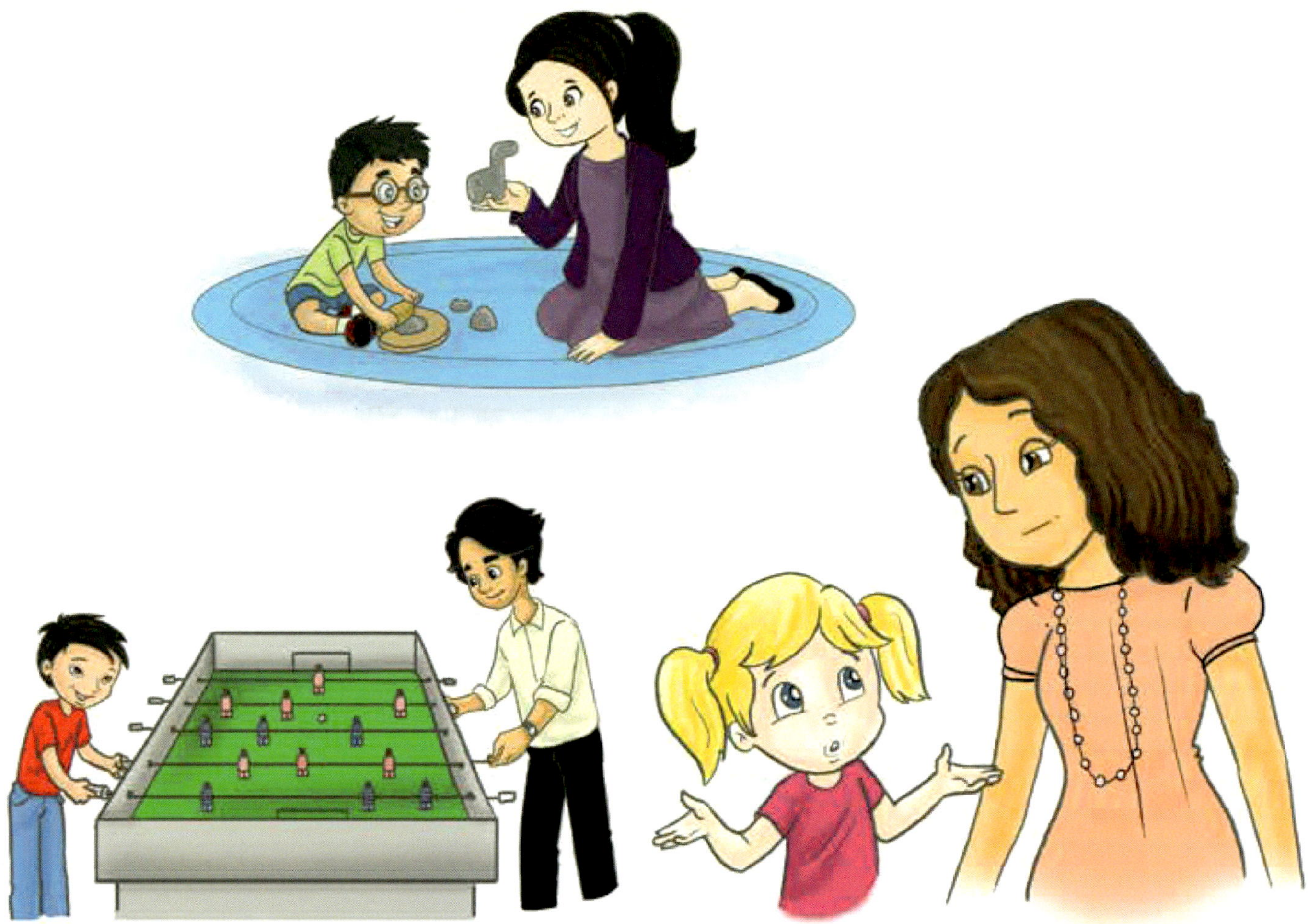

We all had different counselors.

The more we allowed ourselves to talk about the voices, the better we felt.

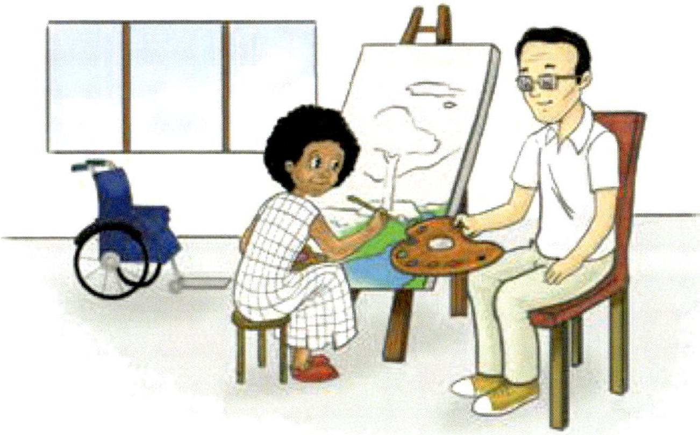

Our counselors definitely helped us a lot.

Each of our counselors helped us understand our voice(s) better.

They explained that often, voices are there for different reasons; sometimes to protect us and at other times to distract, help or express our feelings, experiences and concerns. There can also be other roles for voices in kids' lives.

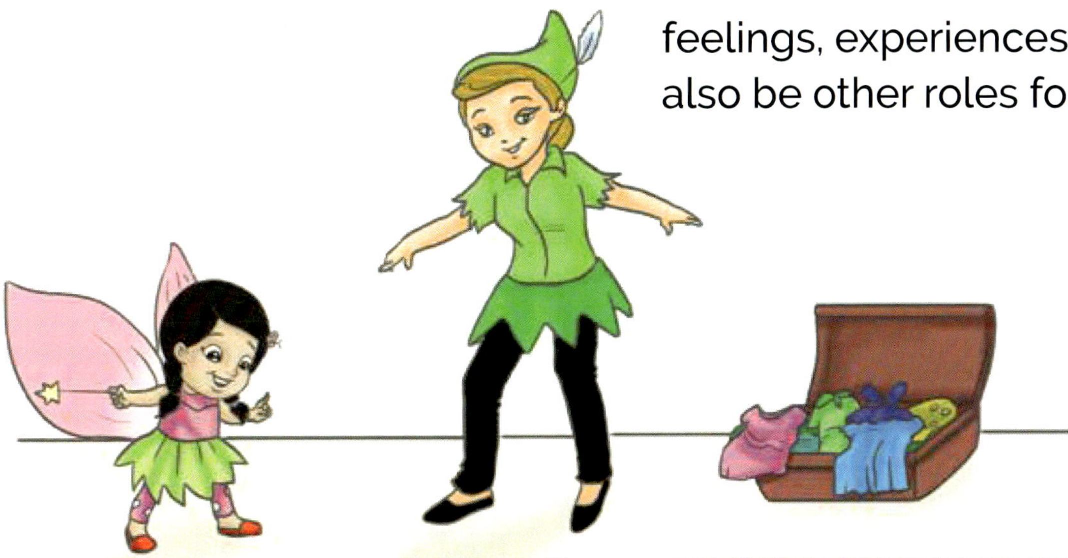

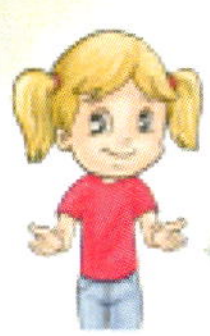

Would you like to know what else we found helpful? Turn the page if you would like to hear the rest of our stories.

After several weeks of talking to Amy, I realized that the voice I heard had something to do with a really bad experience I had when I was younger.

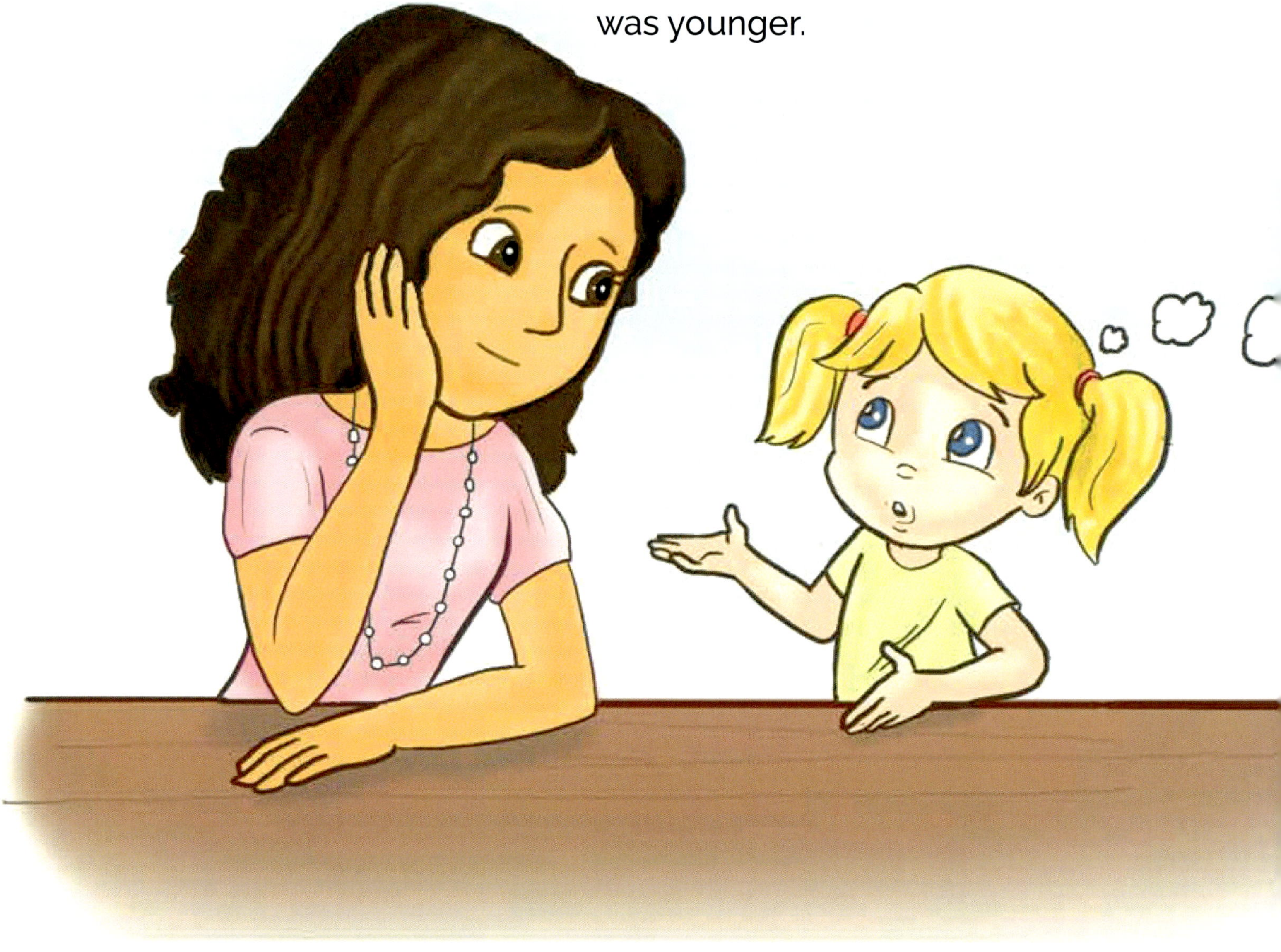

When I was 7 years old, my biological dad used to hit and badly beat me up. This usually happened when he was drunk or, sometimes, even when he was just angry or upset about something.

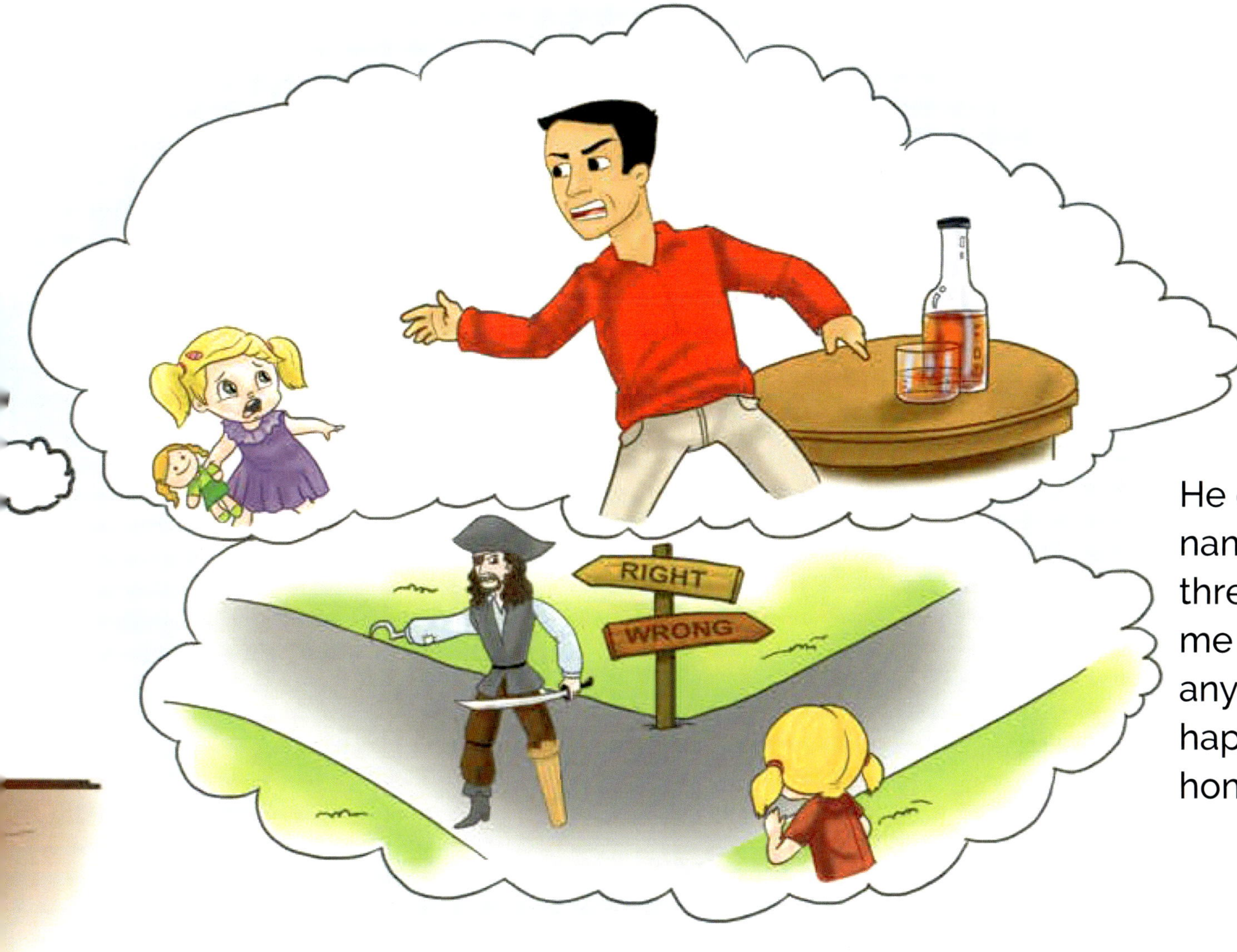

He called me names and threatened to hurt me if I ever told anyone what happened at home.

Although dad does not live with me anymore, what he did to me left me feeling bad for a long time. I held it all in and tried to forget about it but it continued to trouble me.

When my dad was no longer in my life, the one-legged pirate appeared and slowly started to torment me.

After sharing my experience with Amy, I **felt better**.

I learned that the pirate was trying to protect me. Because mistakes used to get me in trouble with my dad, the one-legged pirate tried to make sure I always did the right thing. But he used mean ways to do this.

Even after I figured this out with Amy's help, the one-legged pirate still came around to bother me, although less frequently.

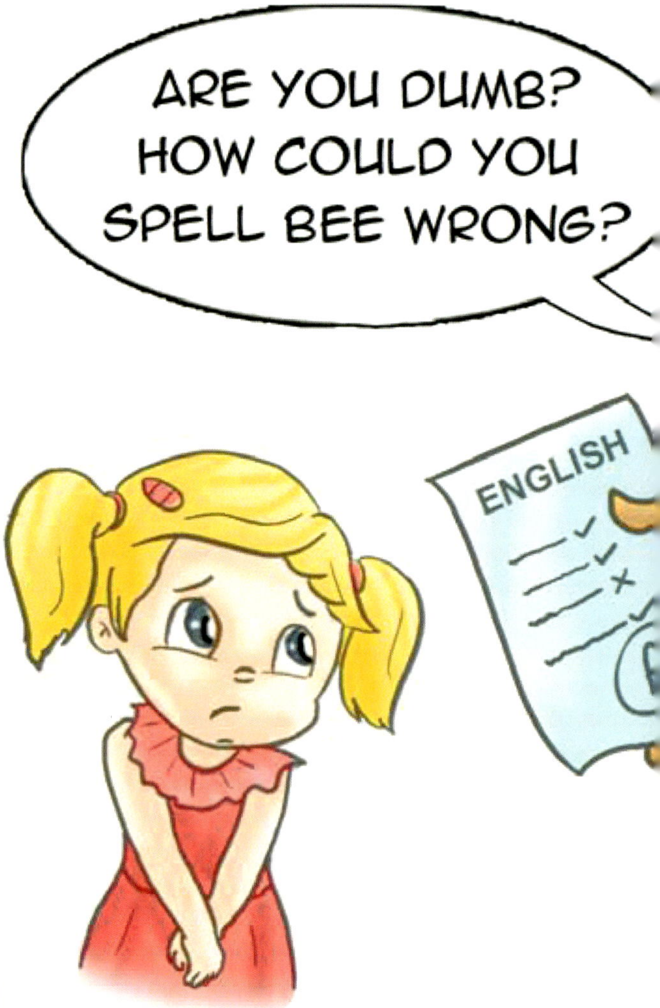
ARE YOU DUMB? HOW COULD YOU SPELL BEE WRONG?
ENGLISH

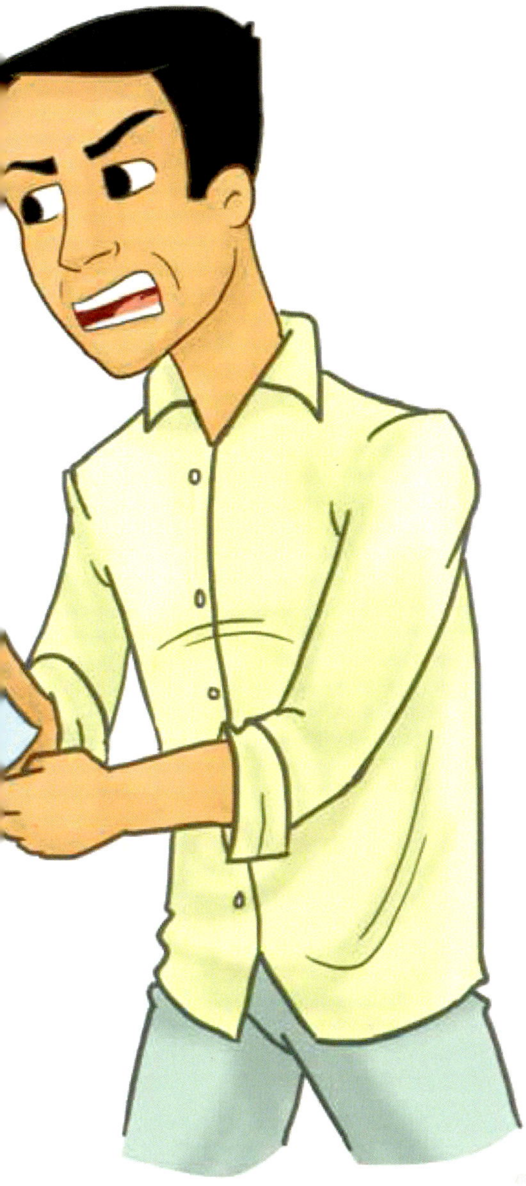

I told Amy I still wanted the one-legged pirate to disappear completely.

We brainstormed to see how I could deal with him. Some ideas we came up with didn't work and others did. I like to call the things that worked for me my "TRICKS". I'd like to tell you about them.

Amy helped me realize a few things.

I learned that it is **okay to make mistakes.** "That's how we learn, Susie. Life is all about learning," she said.

"Sometimes bad experiences in life can leave us feeling like we should not try new things. We may worry about making the perfect decision."

I also realized that what my dad did to me was wrong. Adults have the right to teach and guide young kids like us, but they are not allowed to be abusive.

When adults behave in abusive ways it is usually because they have a problem, like an alcohol problem or an anger problem.

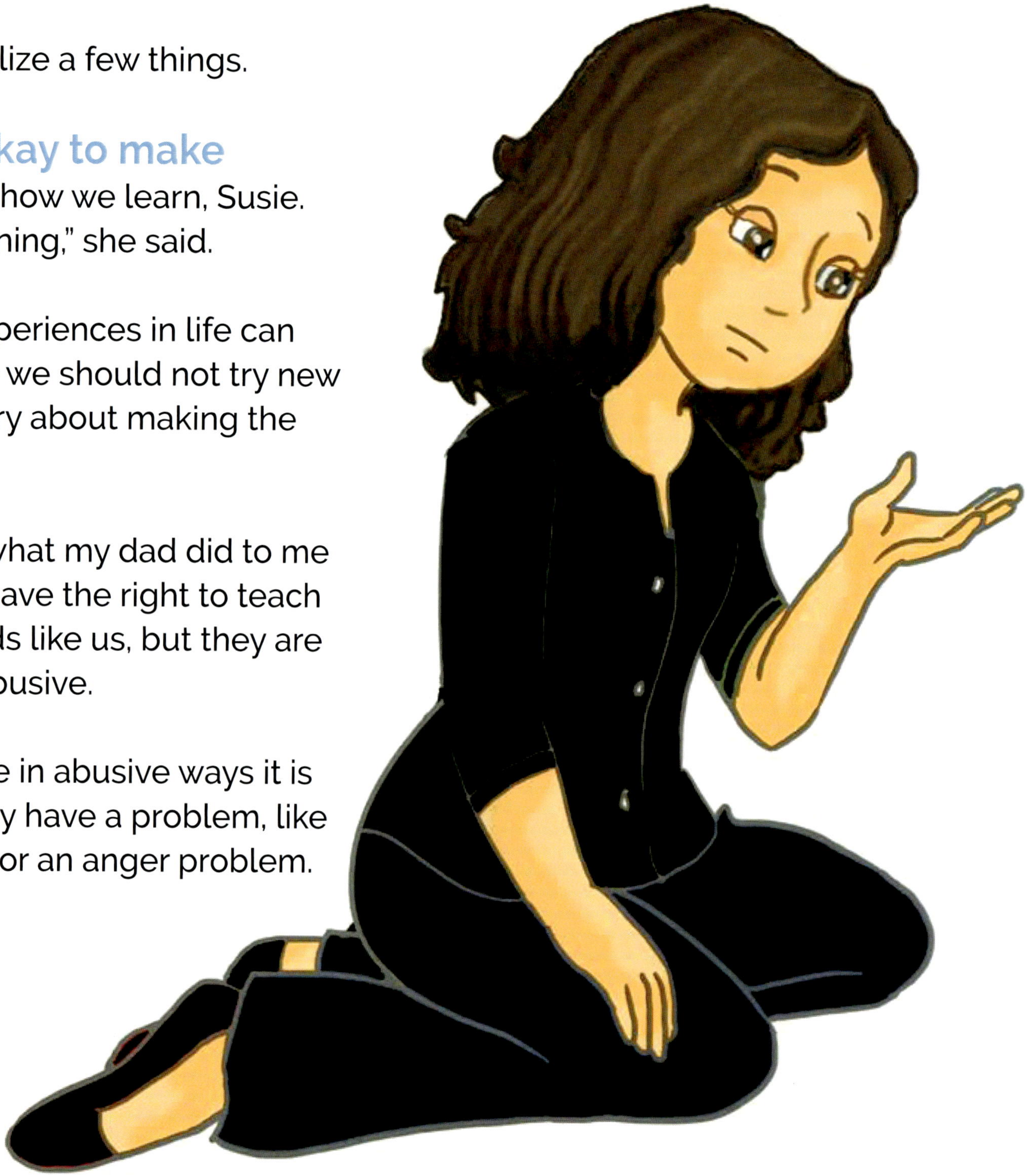

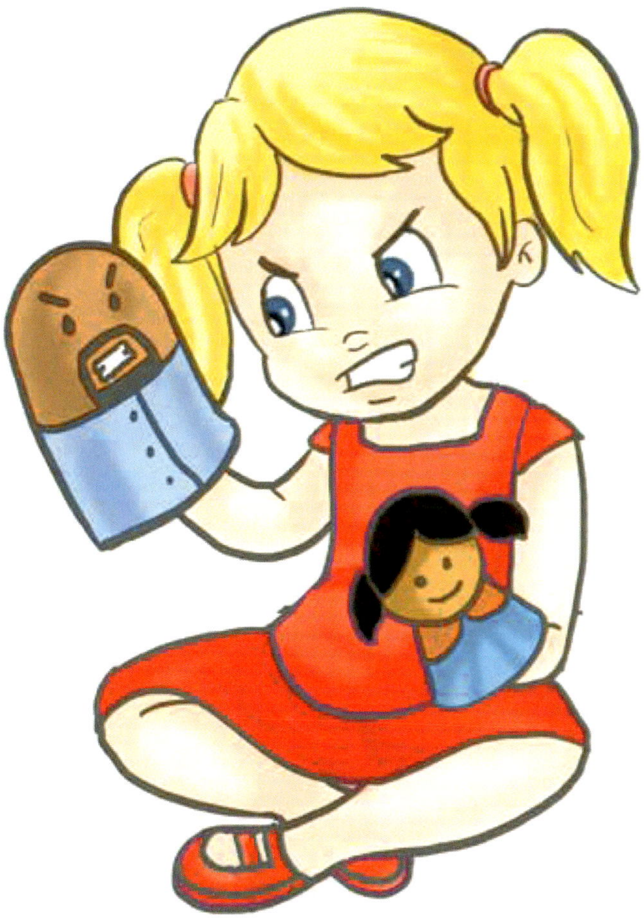

But still it does not make it okay for them to be mean to children.

Amy also told me it is **okay to feel angry** when we are badly treated. Anger is just one of the many feelings human beings have.

Thanks to my counselor, I learned about what to do with my feelings.

These days, I am no longer so angry at my dad. I am also not so angry with the one-legged pirate anymore. They both have problems, but that does not mean that I have to suffer. No one should be treated in such a mean way.

During one of my sessions with Amy, I decided that I wasn't going to allow the pirate to rule my life.

So Amy and I put our heads together.

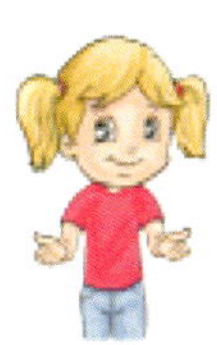

What would you like to do with your voice(s)?
Manage them?
Have them around?
Get rid of them completely?

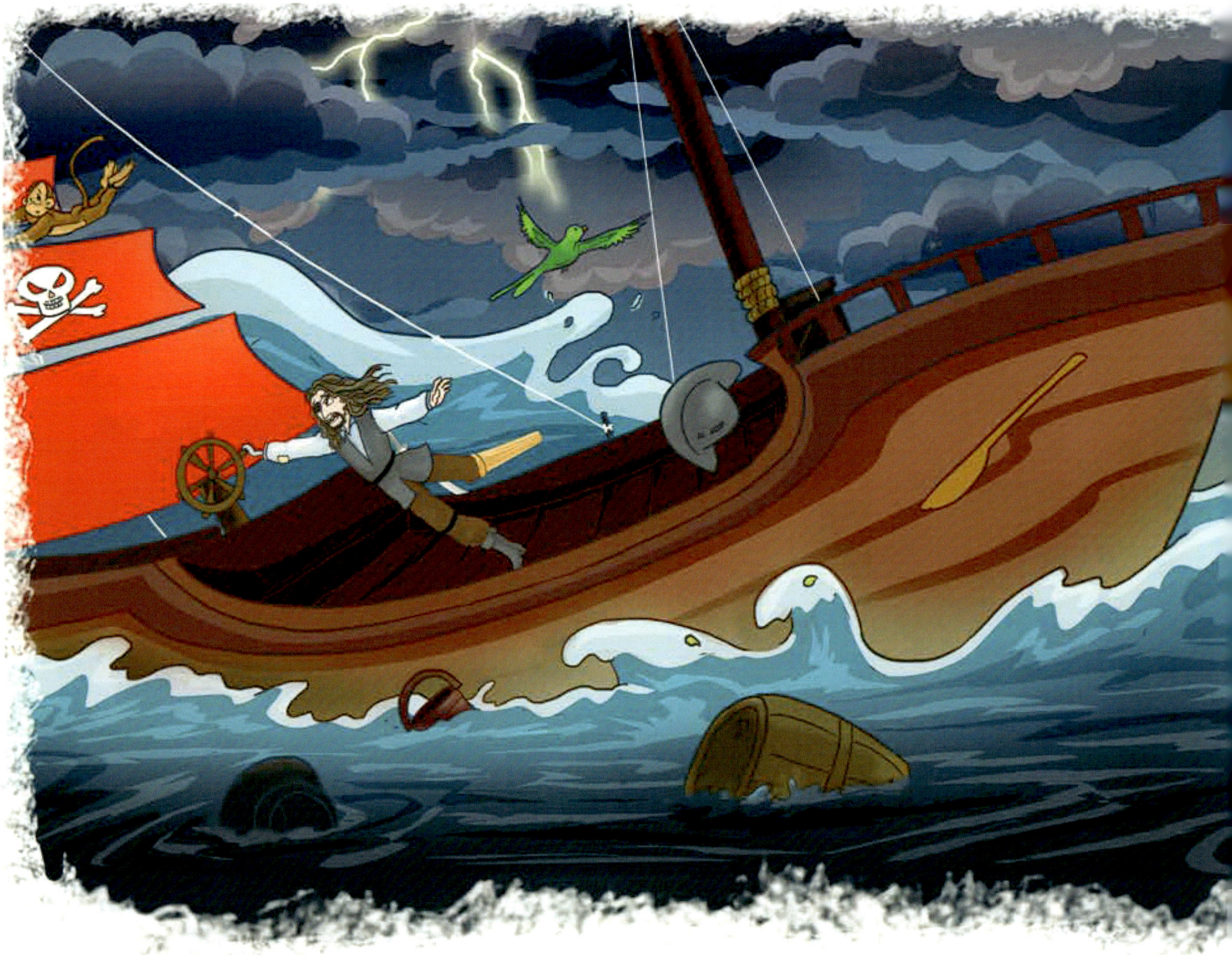

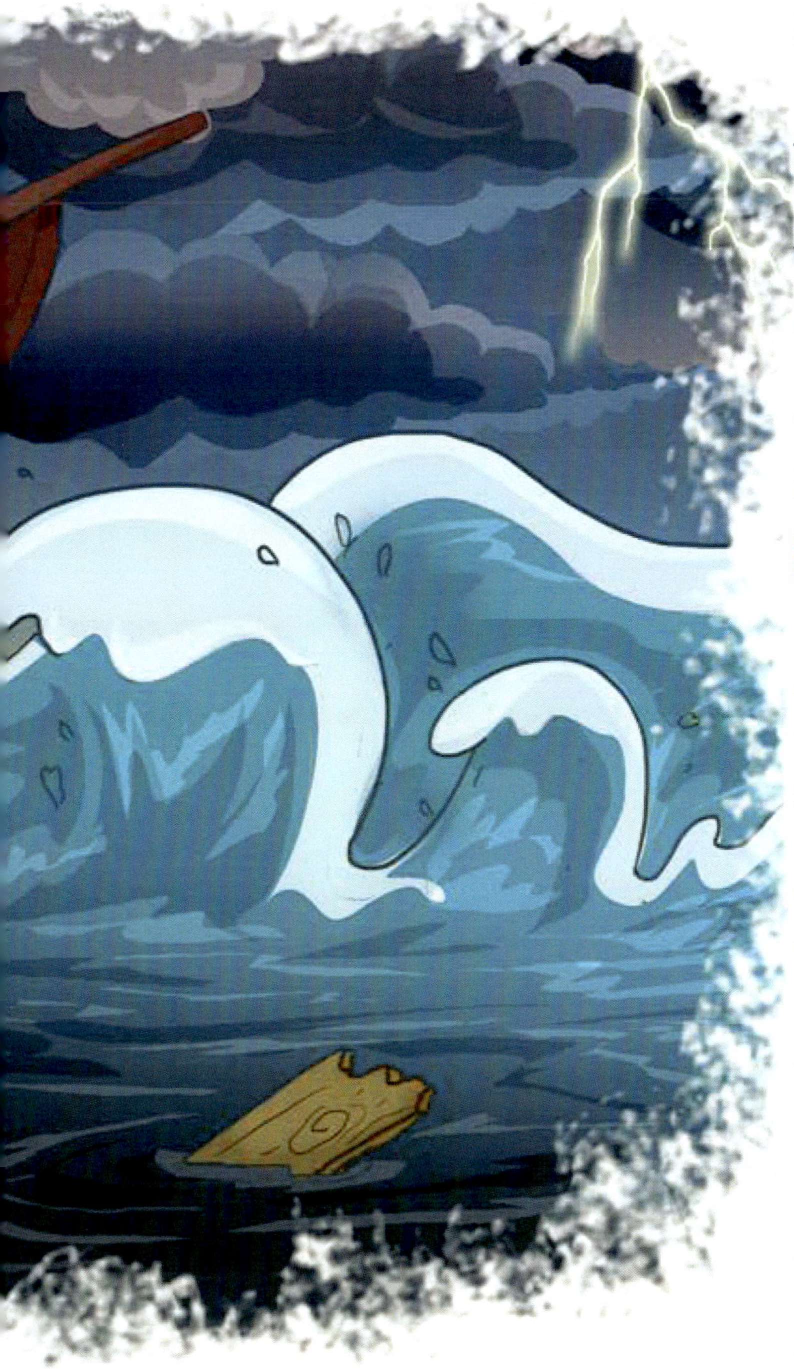

I am so excited that I now get to share with you the **TRICKS** that worked for me!

When the one-legged pirate bullied me, I told him to go pick on someone his own size.

When he threatened to hurt me, I imagined there was a terrible ocean storm with **howling** wind that **ROCKED** his ship so hard he could barely hold on. He would run from one side of the ship to the other, shrieking.

"**Ohhh...No, ohhhh-ohhhh-ohhhh... Yikes!** I can't hold on!"

The storm trick worked when I wanted the one-legged pirate to stop singing too.

After all that rocking and being tossed about, the one-legged pirate couldn't even think about talking, let alone singing annoying pirate songs.

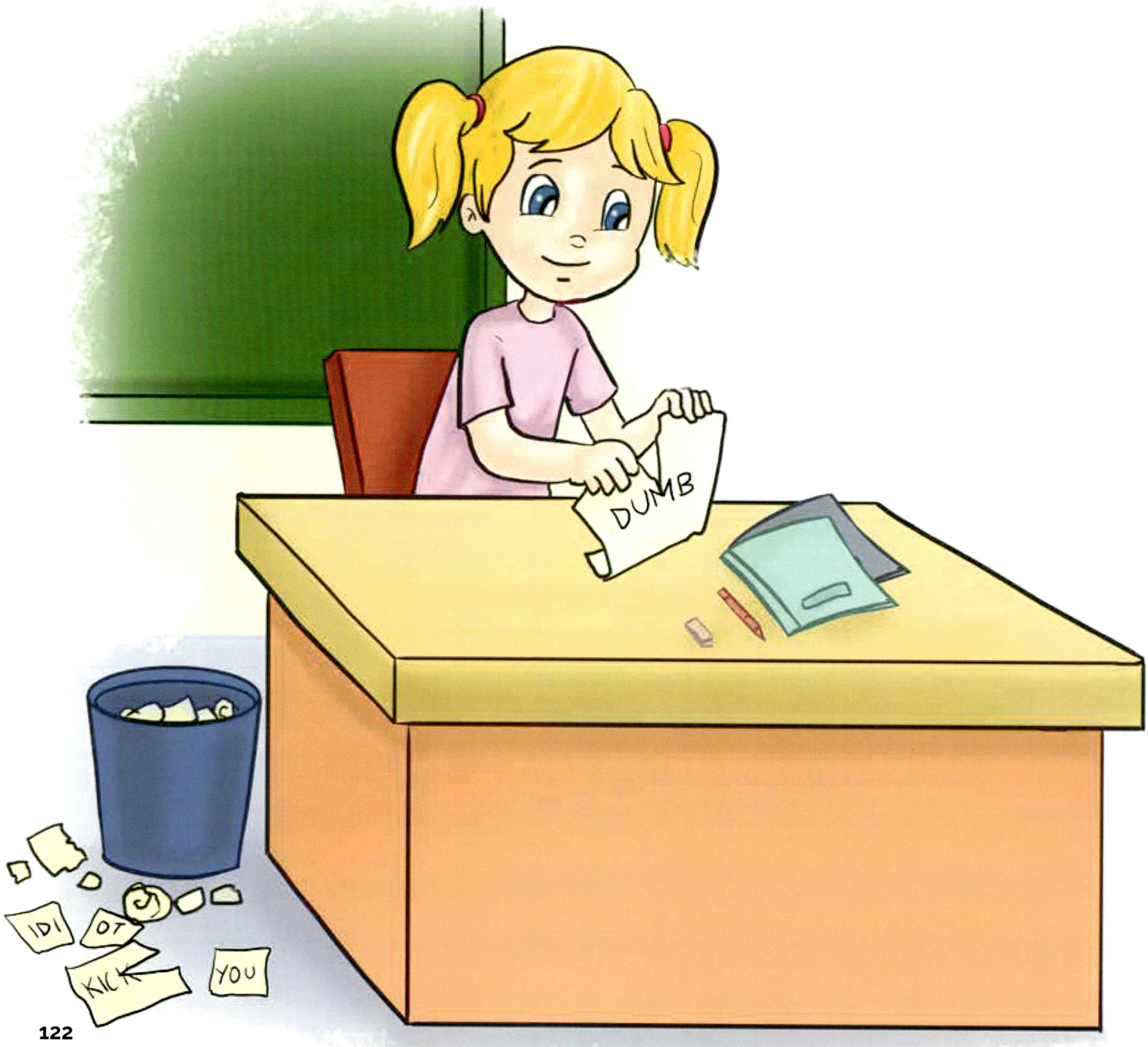
DUMB
IDI
OT
KICK
YOU

If I needed to focus on schoolwork and the one-legged pirate persisted in bugging me, I wrote out the words and names he was calling me on a piece of paper. Then I tore it up and threw the bits of paper away.

POOF!!

The one-legged pirate's nasty words were destroyed!

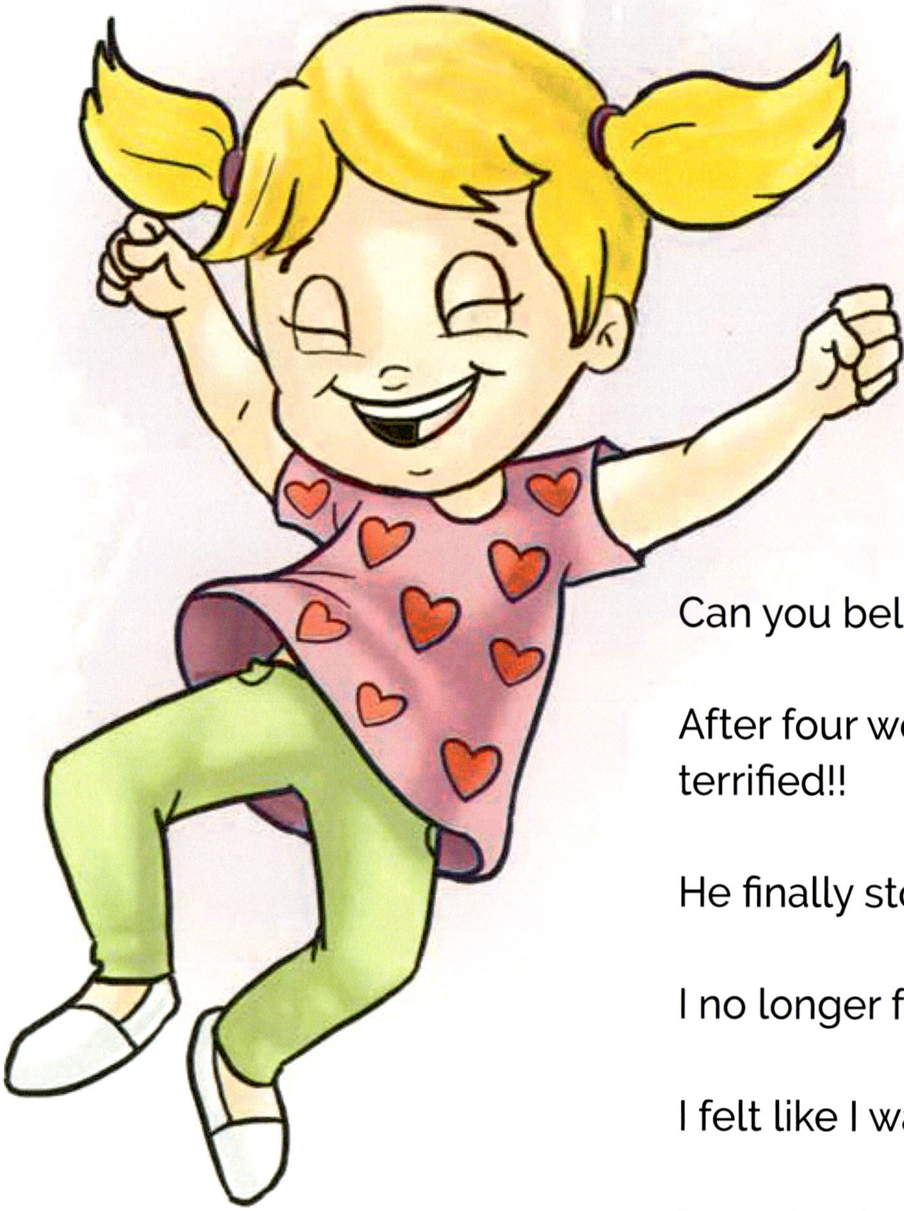

Can you believe it!!?

After four weeks, I didn't feel so afraid and terrified!!

He finally stopped pestering me.

I no longer felt so angry.

I felt like I was in charge.

My schoolwork got better. During exams and tests, I decided when I wanted to listen to him and when I didn't.

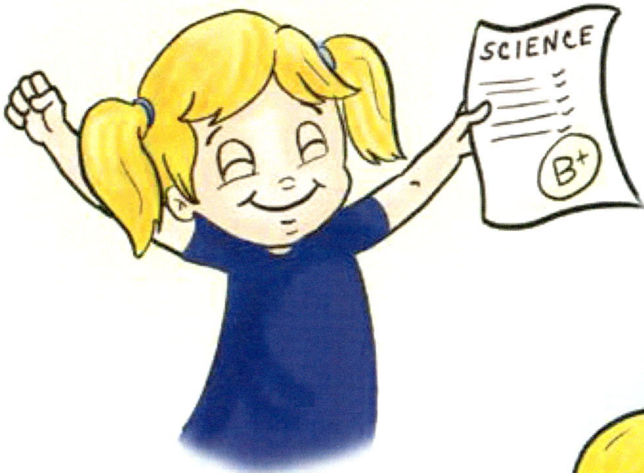

Finally, things changed in my life. I got a B+ in my favorite subject, science.

My schoolwork got better in general. I started making friends at school and Mr Jones, my teacher, was pleased with my improvements.

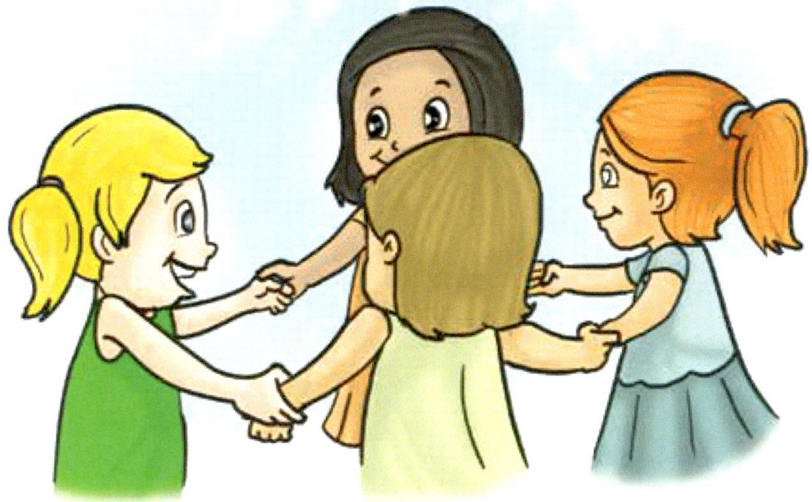

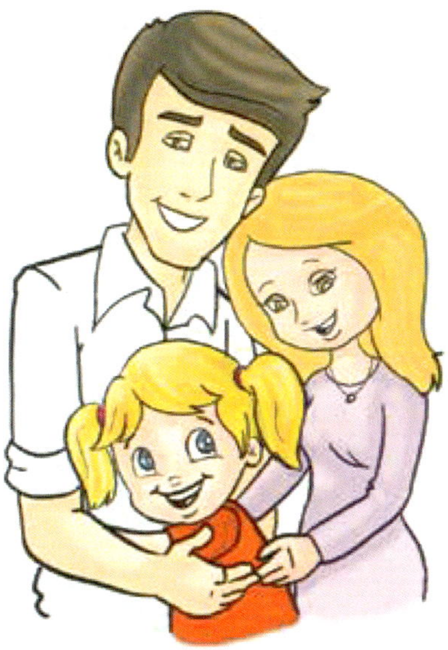

My parents were **ecstatic!** I was so **proud** of myself!

I couldn't believe it! **I DID IT!**

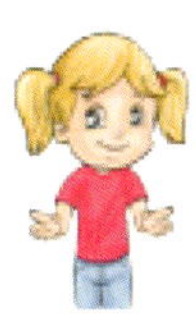

Have you ever felt proud of yourself? When? What about?
Do you want to know what happened with the voices that Carlos and the others heard? Go on, flip the page.

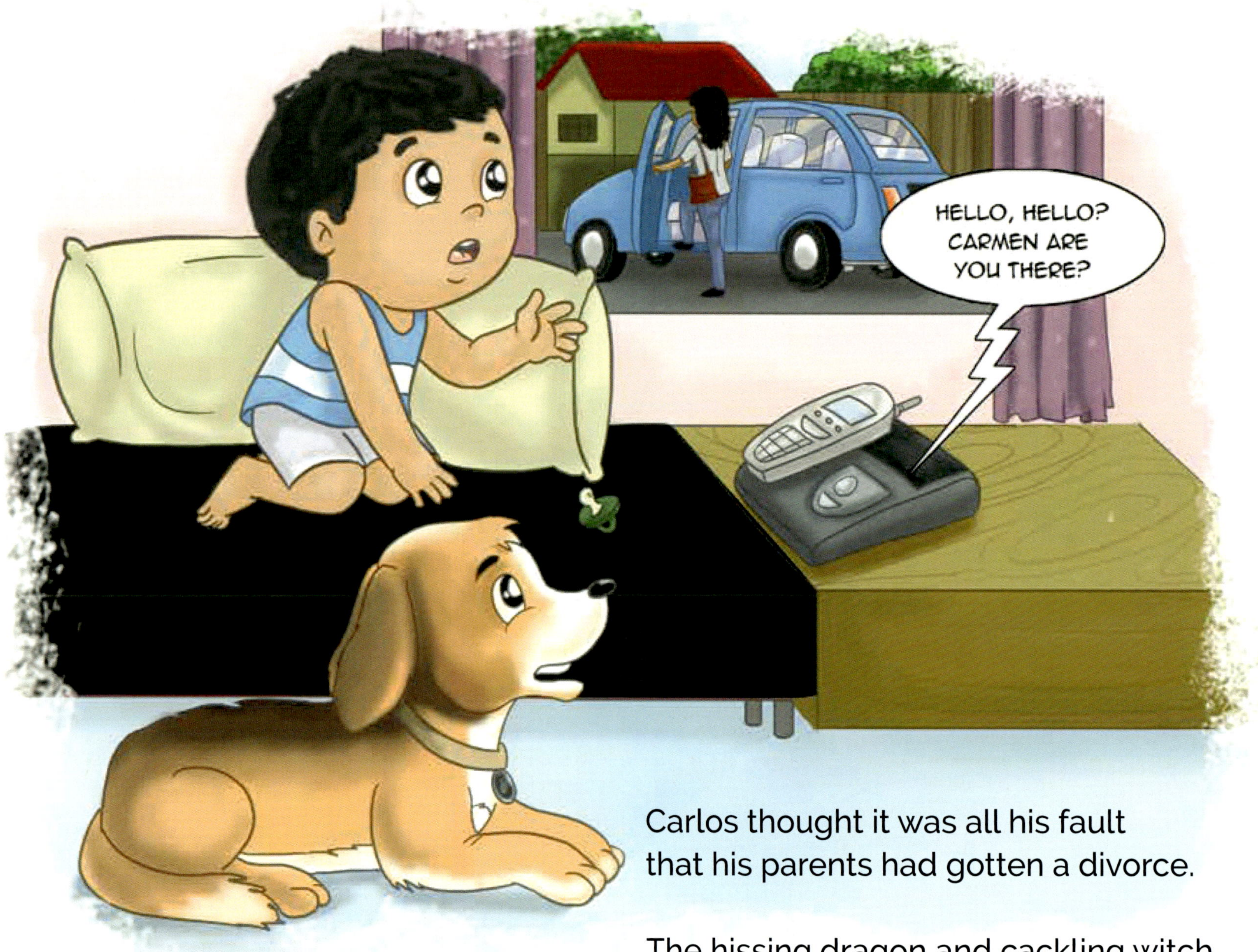

Carlos thought it was all his fault that his parents had gotten a divorce.

The hissing dragon and cackling witch came about right around the time of his parents' separation.

Carlos' counselor helped him understand that parents divorce for adult reasons that have nothing to do with their children.

Carlos also discovered that parents are supposed to make sure children are taken care of, and what his mother did was not right.

His mother frequently left him alone at home when he was too young to take care of himself.

Sometimes he felt bored and alone and at other times he felt sad and scared. He cried a lot when he was younger.

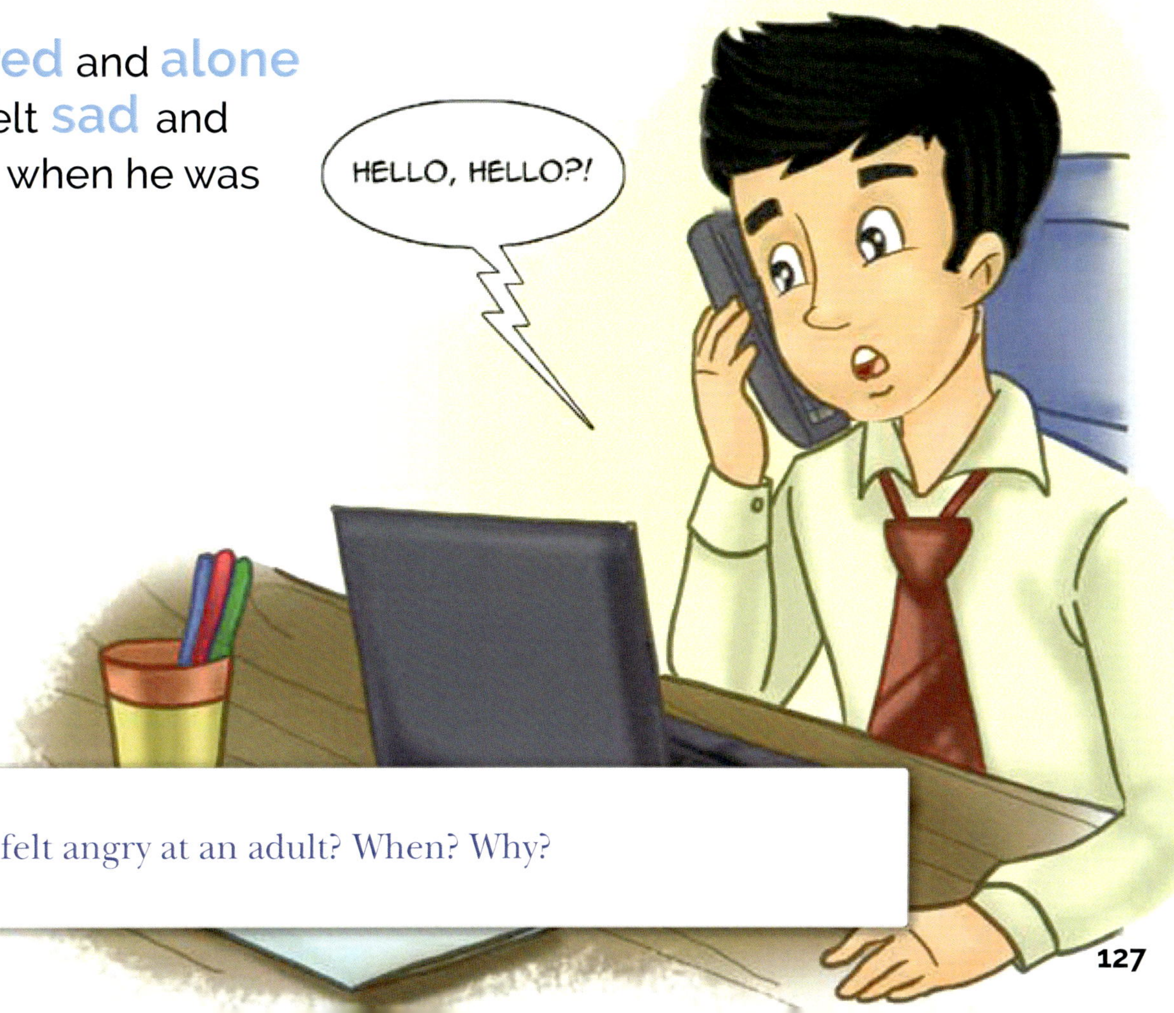

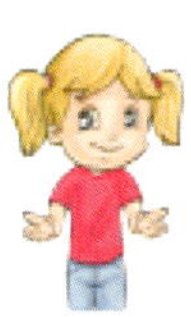

Have you ever felt angry at an adult? When? Why?

When Carlos' dad attended one of his counseling sessions, he told Carlos he was very sorry that he was not cared for the way he should have been.

He said that his mom had problems and that is why she had a hard time caring for Carlos the way she should have.

Carlos felt very **depressed** when he heard this.

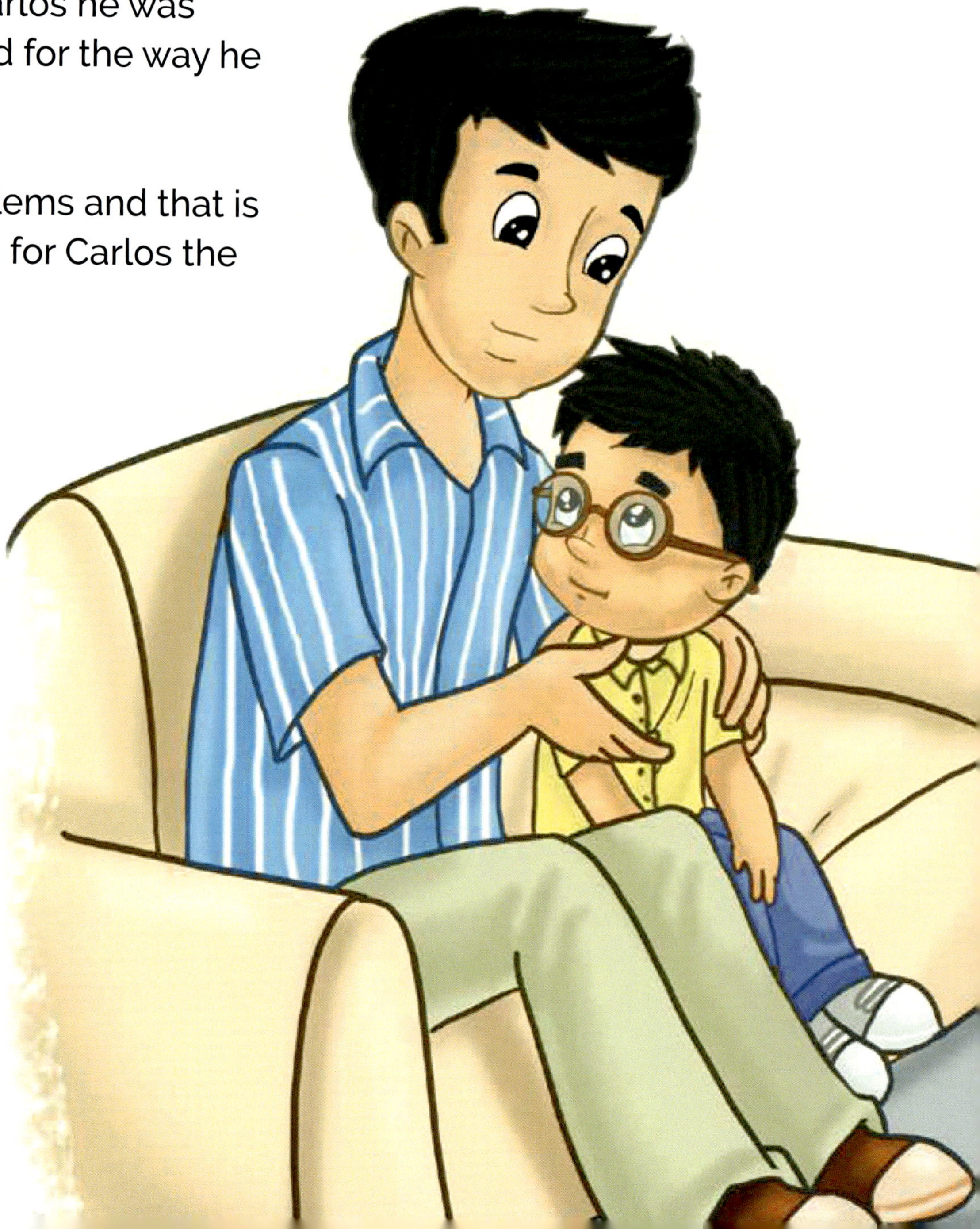

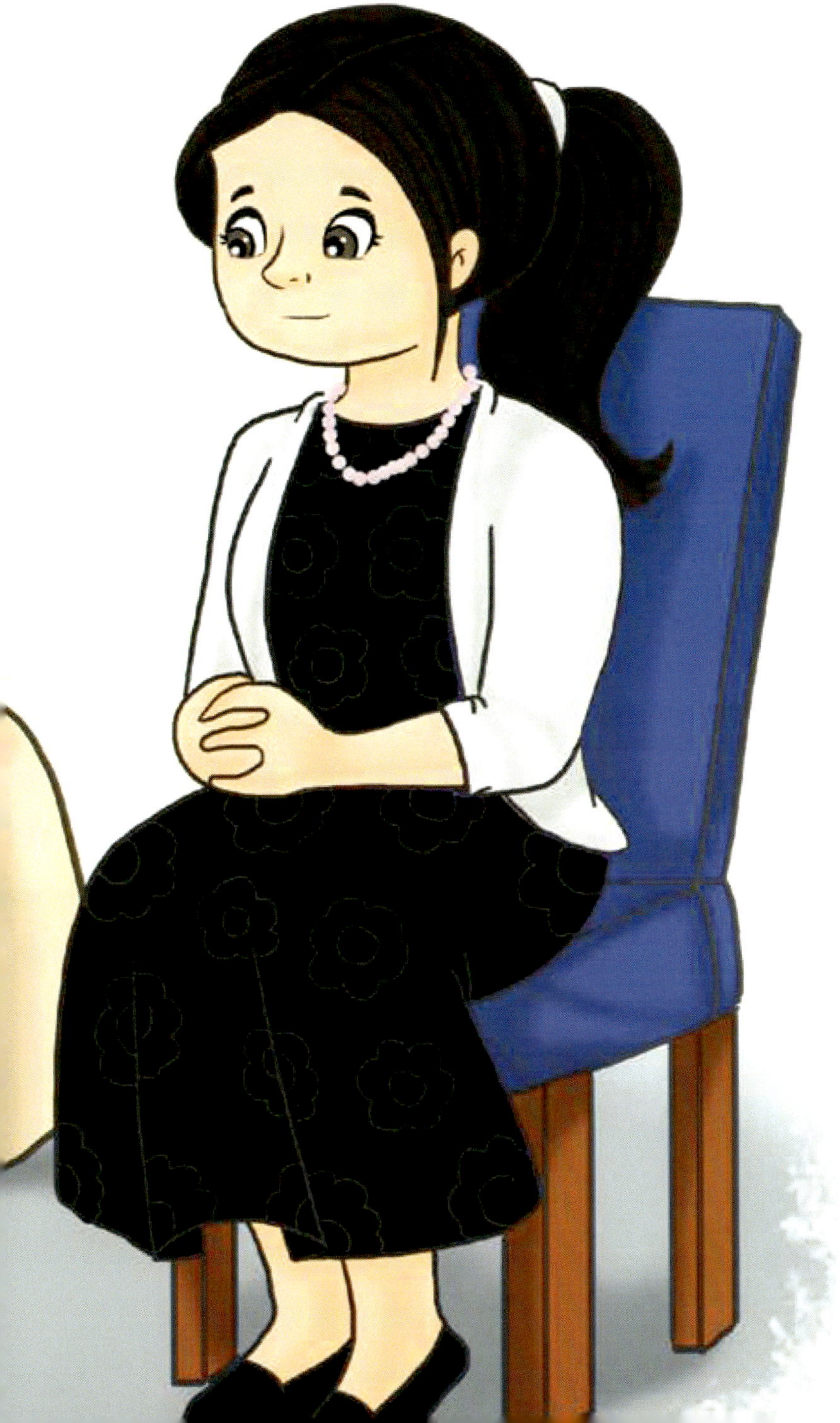

Later, Carlos and his counselor started to talk about how it is **okay** for kids **to feel sad, upset, mad,** and even **disappointed** with their parents or adults when they are not taken care of.

Carlos' counselor explained that because kids are not adults, they need parents to help take care of them.

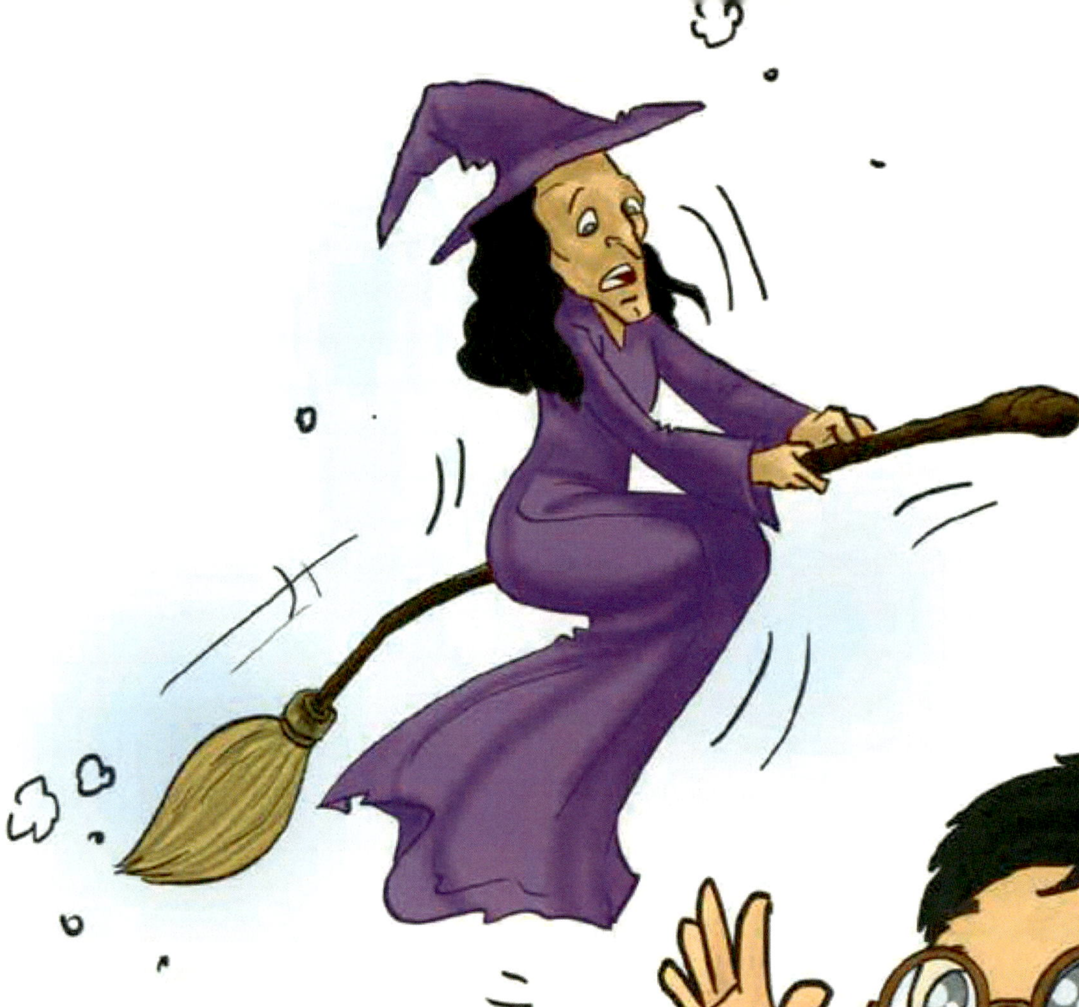

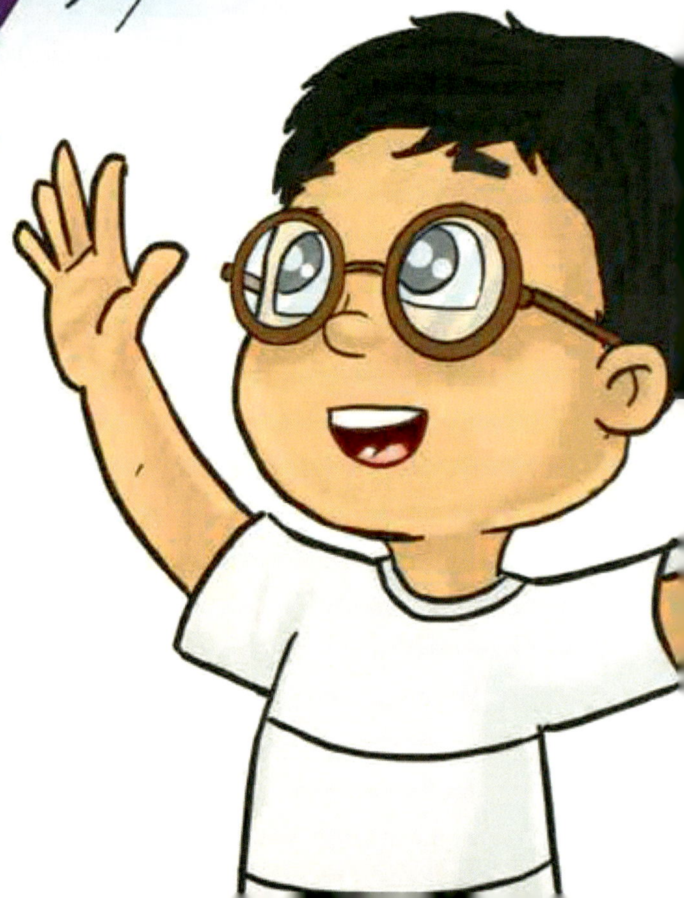

Carlos felt **relieved** to know that divorce does not happen because of children.

He was even more **relieved** to know that it is okay for kids to feel upset with adults or parents.

It felt good to know that there was a reason for his voices and why they were so hot and angry.

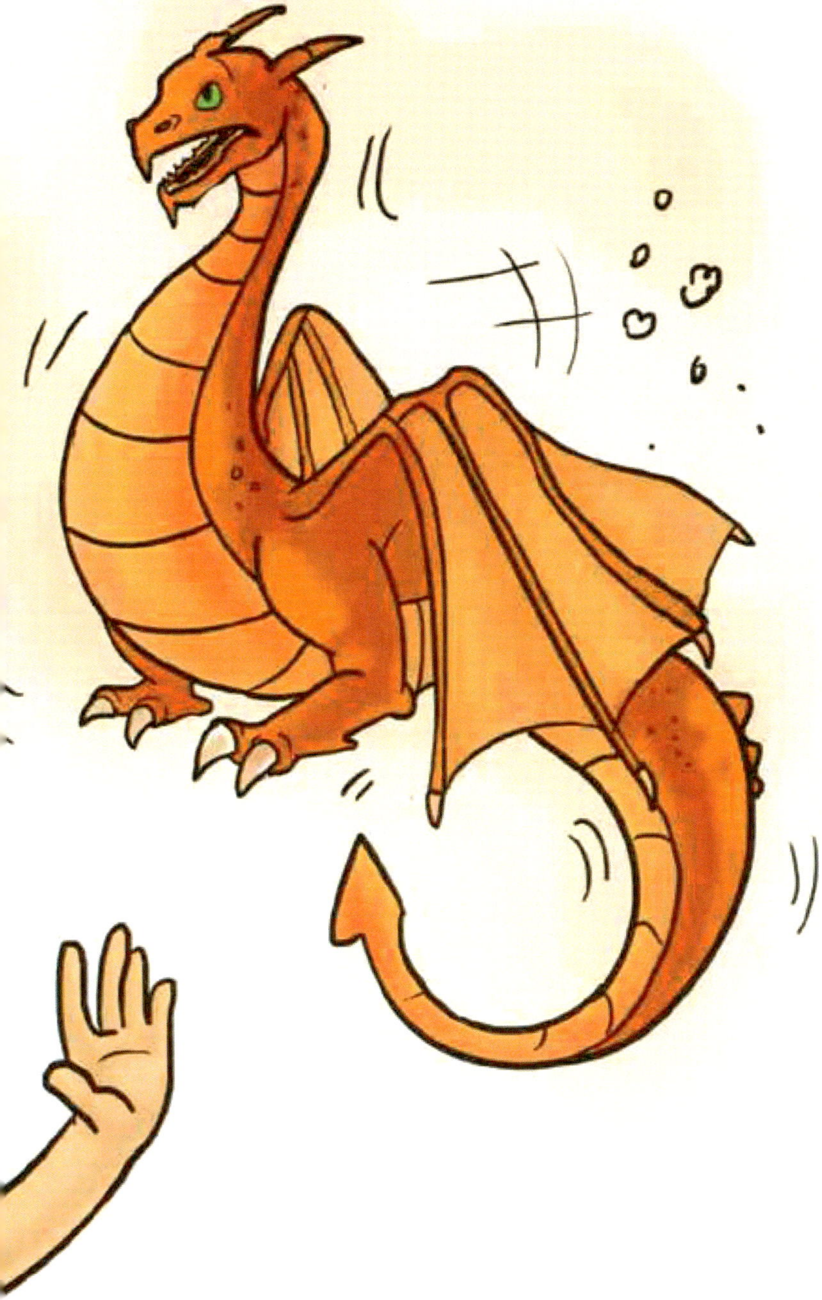

Carlos knew he was not crazy.

He realized he was a good person who experienced all sorts of feelings, including angry feelings.

He understood that his voices were trying to protect him from feeling uncomfortable and sometimes scary emotions like anger, sadness, and fear.

As he felt more comfortable with experiencing and dealing with these sorts of feelings, the voices became less scary. They just became a part of life and his life got better.

When Carlos felt the dragon and the witch were too much to handle, he used several TRICKS.

One of them was to imagine he had one hand on a dial that controlled the volume of the voices and the other on a switch that could completely turn off the hissing and cackling when he wanted to.

To manage the dragon's extremely hot breath, he imagined throwing ice cold water on it and watched the water fizzle and evaporate away.

For the mean witch, to make her say only sweet things, Carlos poured fresh golden honey on her.

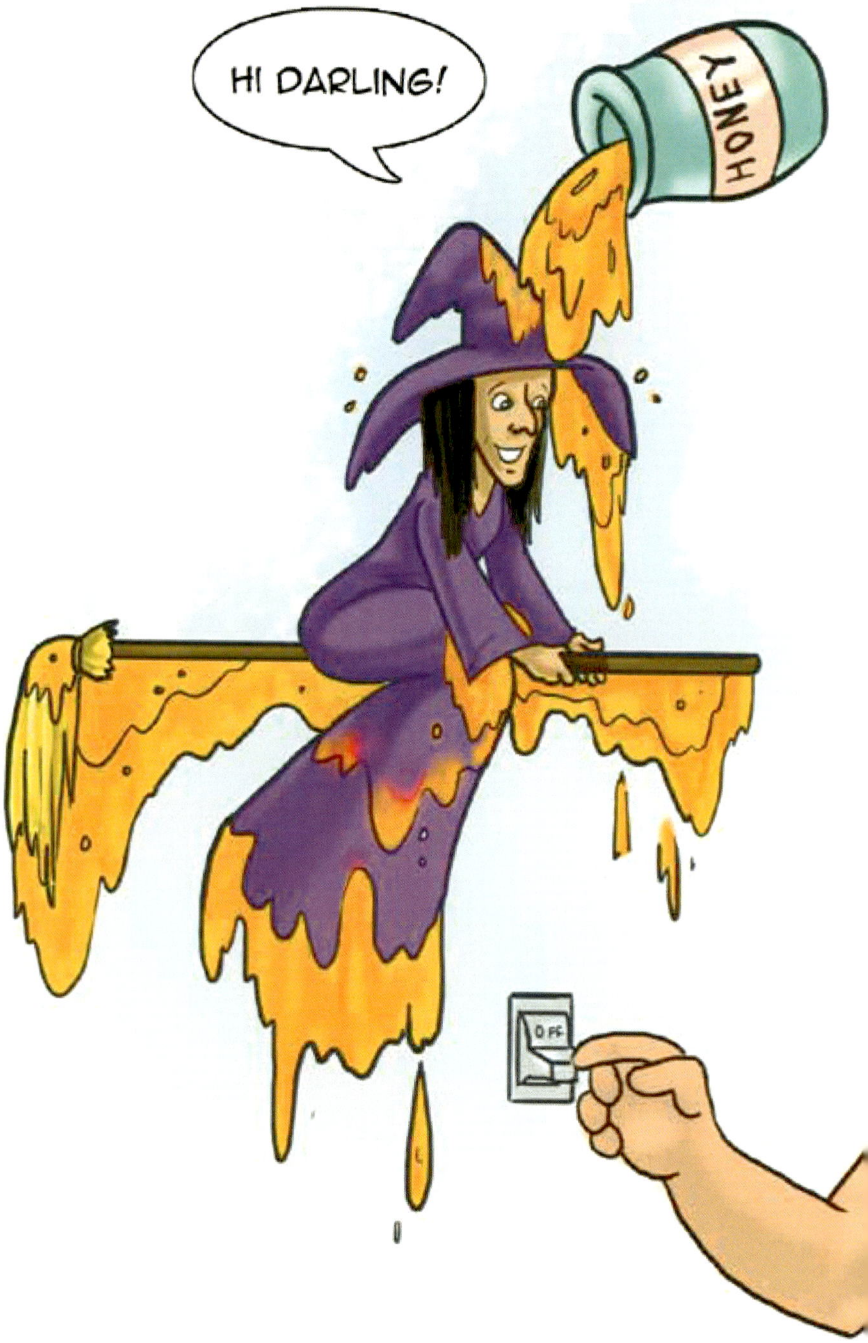

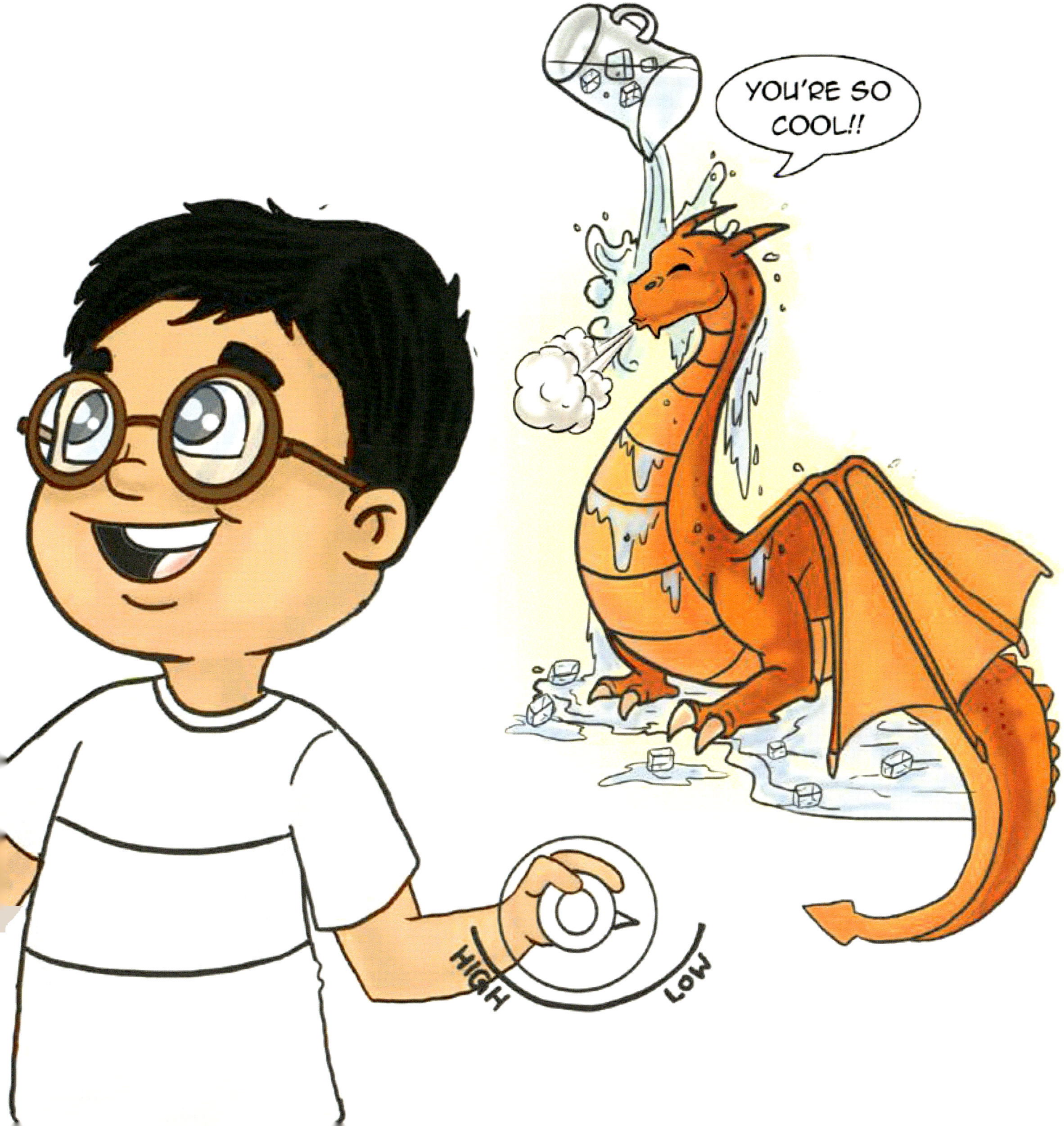
YOU'RE SO
COOL!!
HIGH
LOW

Two weeks later, things got really cool, quiet and sweeter.

Carlos started playing with his friends again.

Carlos no longer felt powerless.

He decided when he gave the voices his attention and when they needed to be quiet.

Carlos kept using his TRICKS.

After some time, the witch and dragon didn't bother him so much.

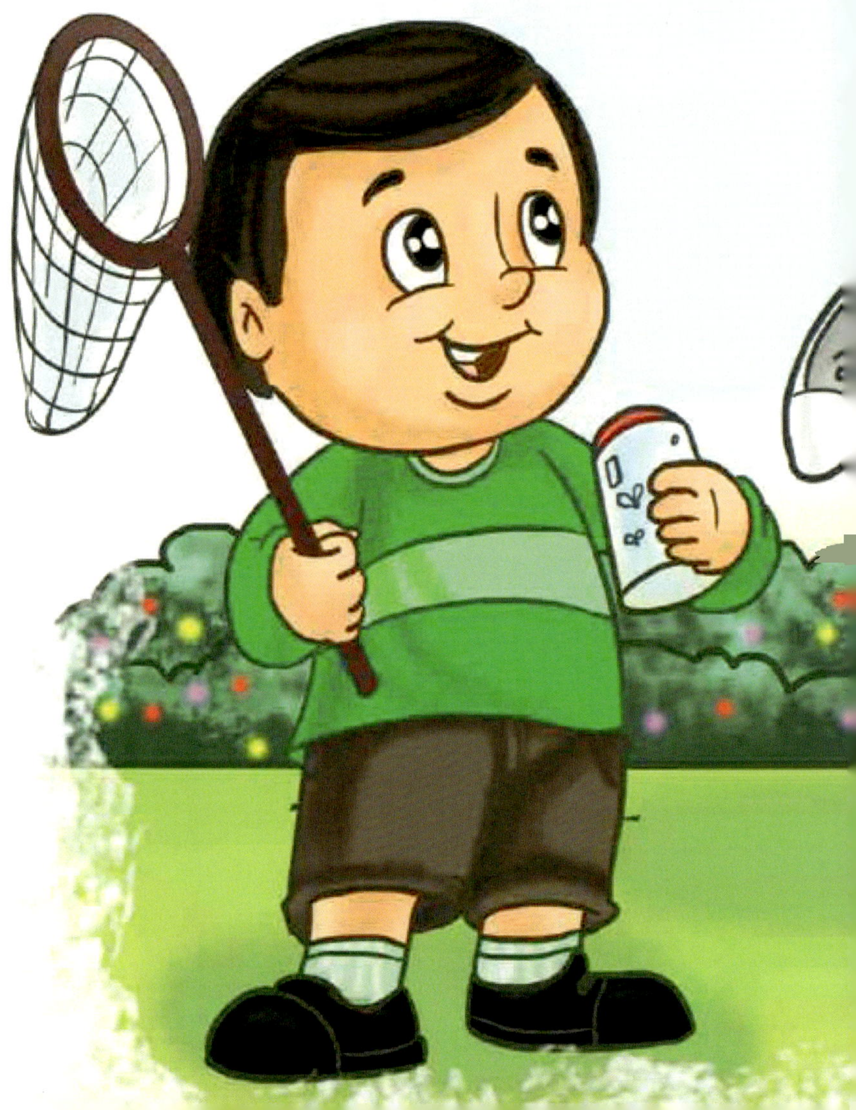

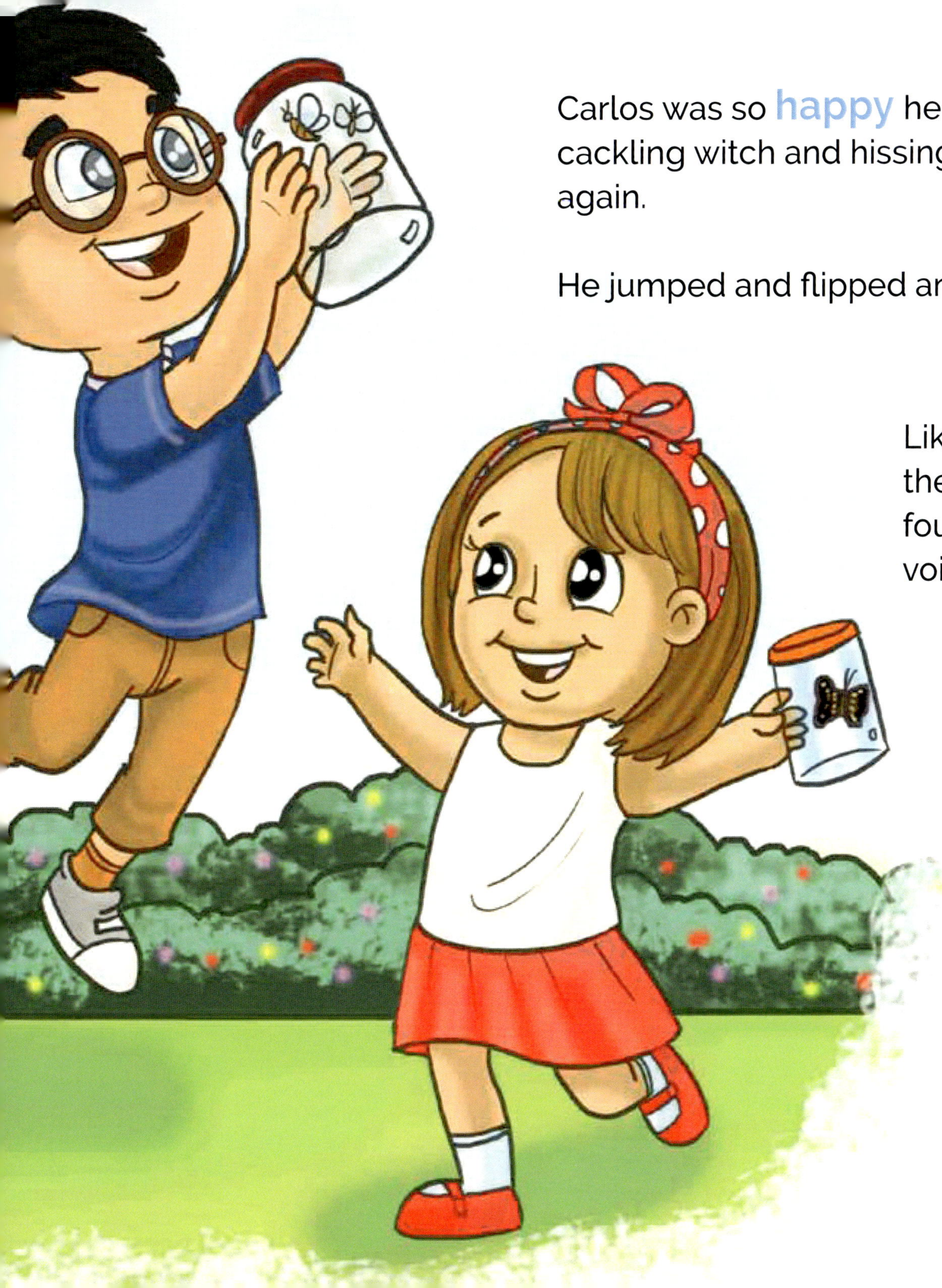

Carlos was so happy he had managed the cackling witch and hissing dragon and life was fun again.

He jumped and flipped and danced!

Like Carlos and I, Chang and the rest of the gang also found ways to manage their voices.

Turn the page to read about their discoveries, TRICKS, tools and experiences.

Let's look at what happened to Selma's three voices.

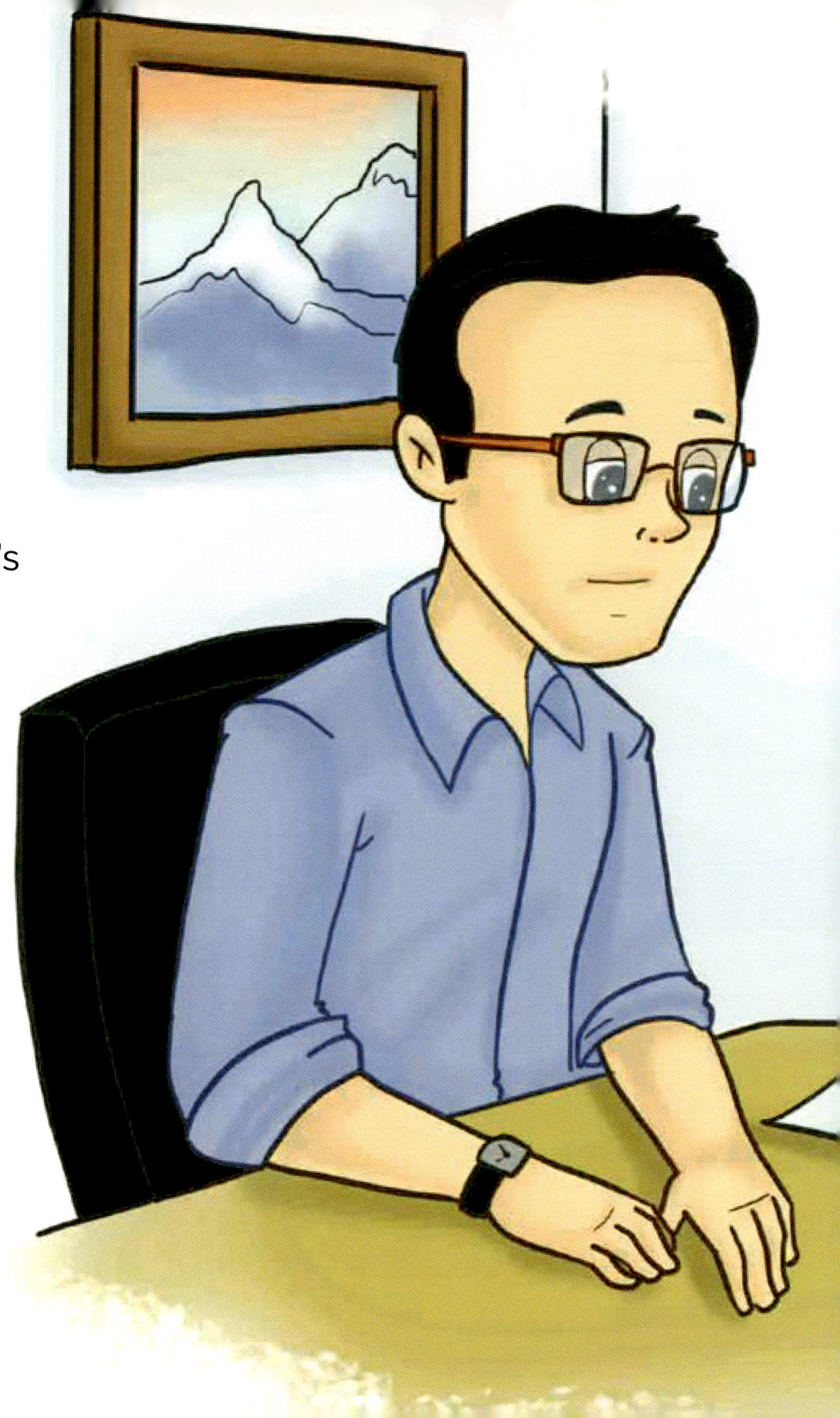

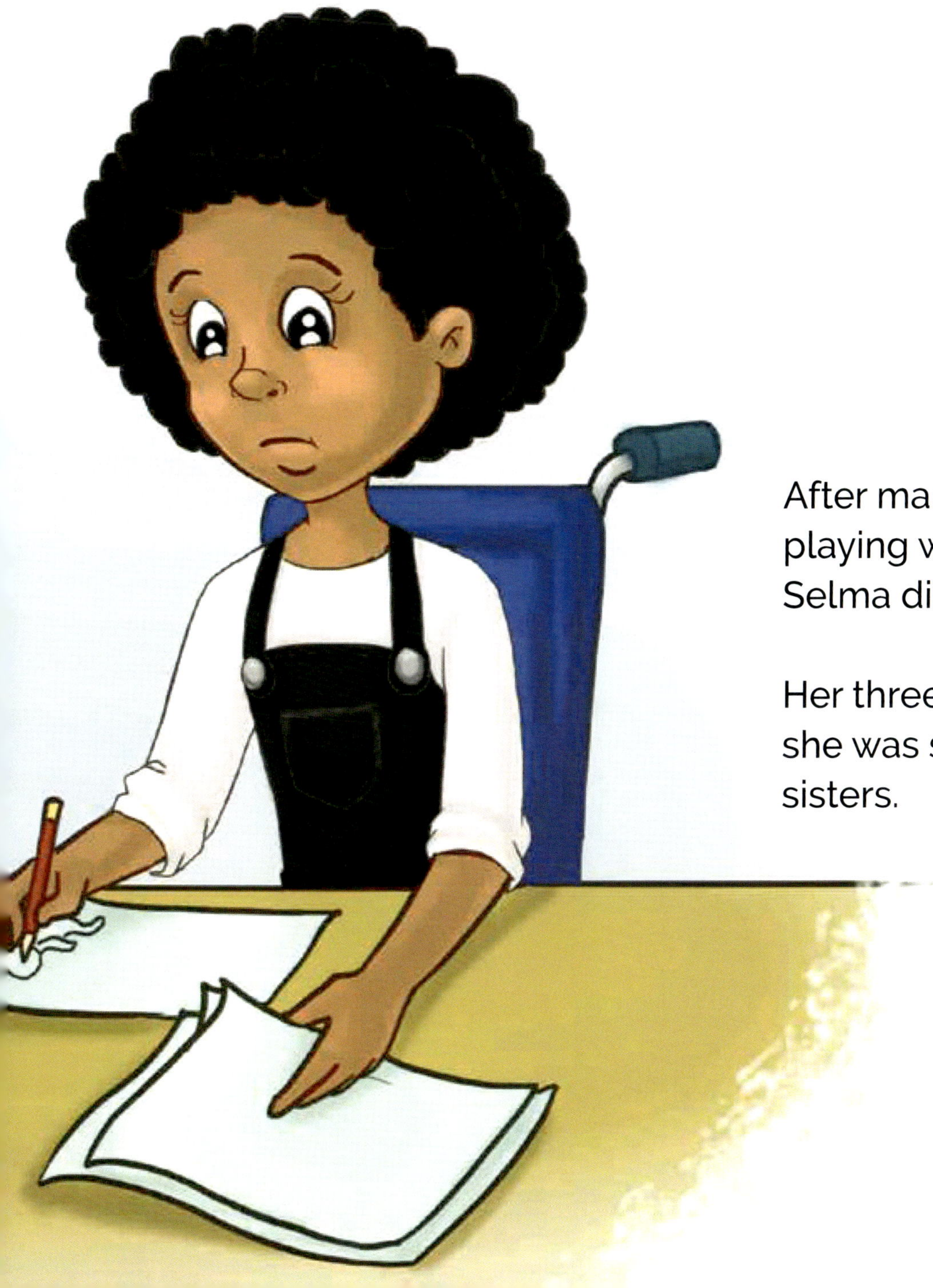

After many weeks of talking, drawing and playing with toys in her counselor's room, Selma discovered something.

Her three voices appeared shortly after she was separated from her two younger sisters.

When Selma was 6 years old, her father had been mean to her and her sisters. He touched all of them in places that made them feel really uncomfortable and bad.

Frequently, Selma tried to protect her sisters from their father but was not always successful.

Finally, Selma's father was not allowed to be around the children. Because Selma's mother could not provide them with the safest place to live, each child was sent to live with a different foster family.

After moving into her foster home, Selma missed her mom, dad and sisters very much.

She often thought it was her fault that her sisters got hurt.

"If only I had stopped dad from hurting my little sisters, Shakira and Shala, we would still be a family," she'd think.

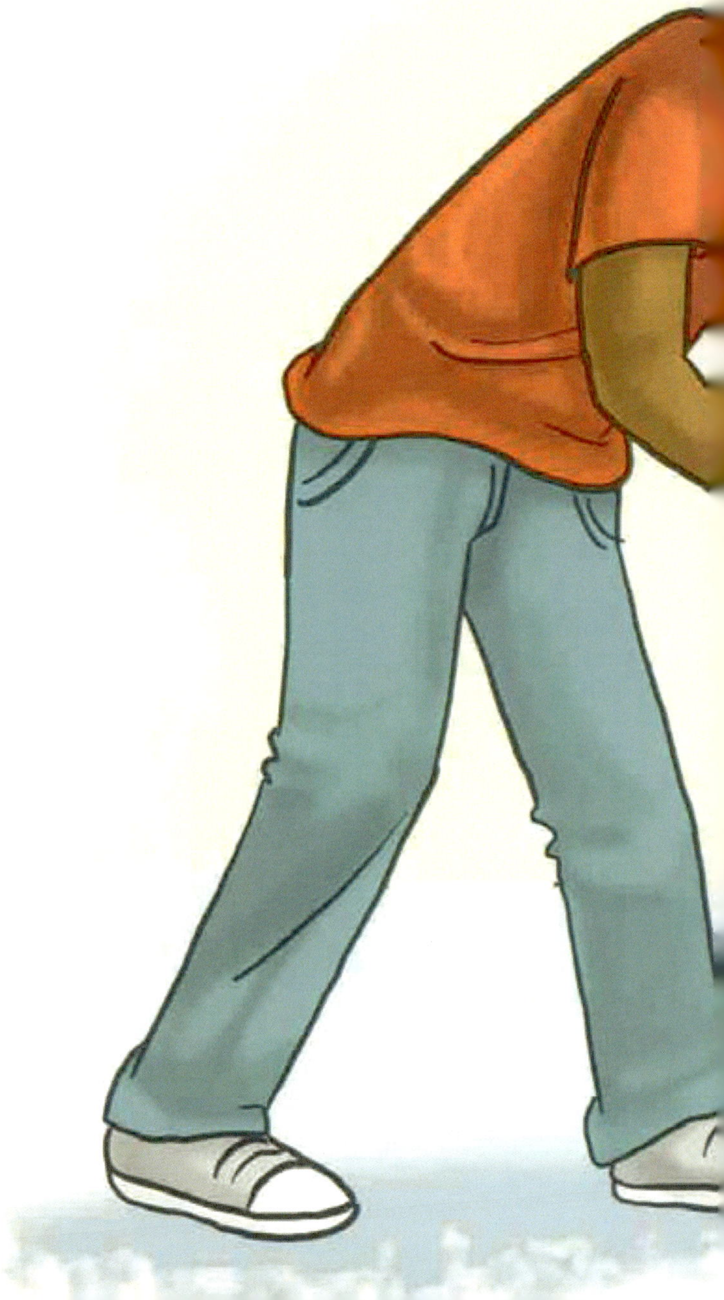

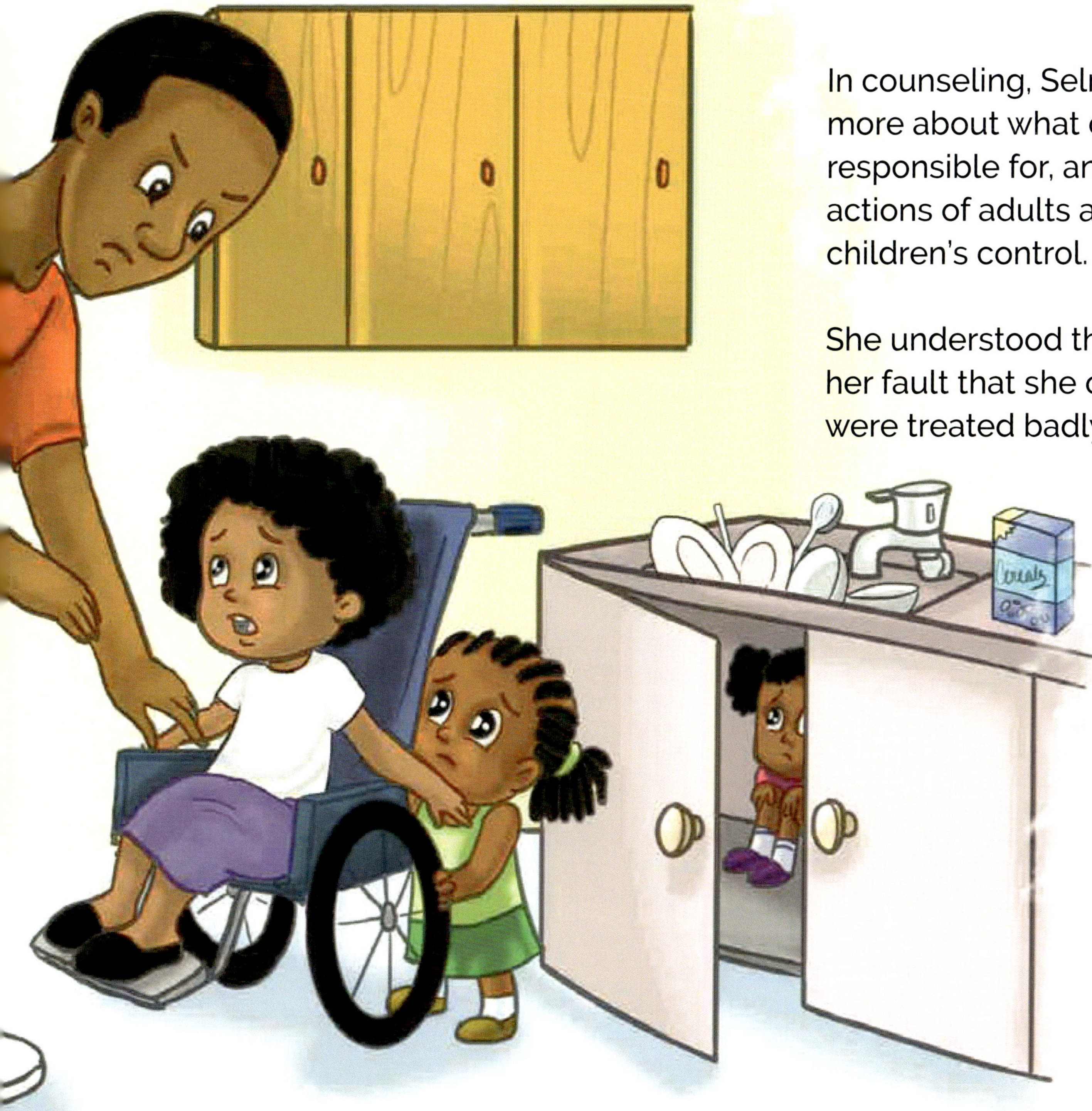

In counseling, Selma learned more about what children are responsible for, and that the actions of adults are not within children's control.

She understood that it was not her fault that she or her sisters were treated badly.

Selma loved her voices, Chuki and Aisha, as much as she loved her biological sisters. She enjoyed the chatter of the voices.

She also realized that it was okay to find them annoying and take breaks from them.

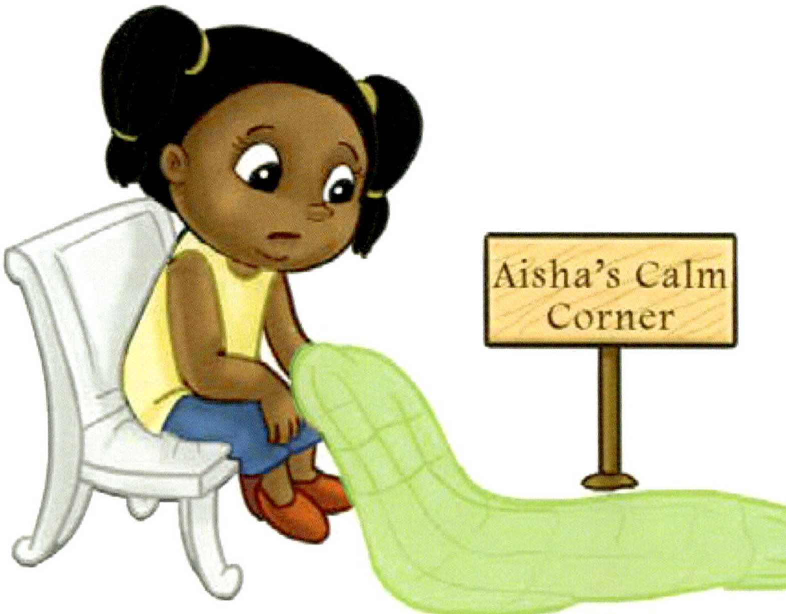

Just as Chuki and Aisha were not her responsibility, protecting her biological sisters was not her responsibility.

She was just a kid herself.

Selma developed a bag of TRICKS that helped her live with her voices.

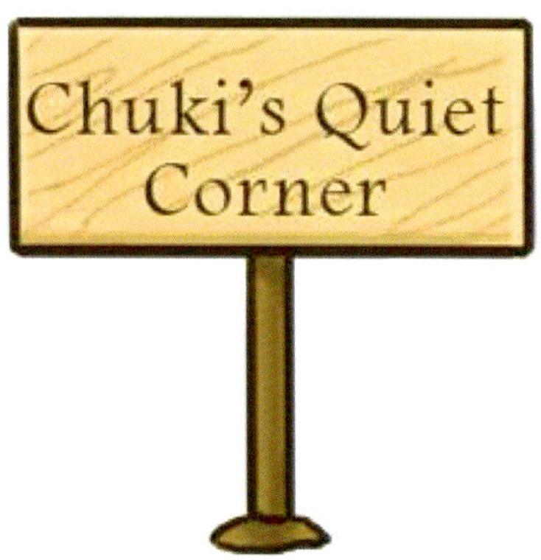

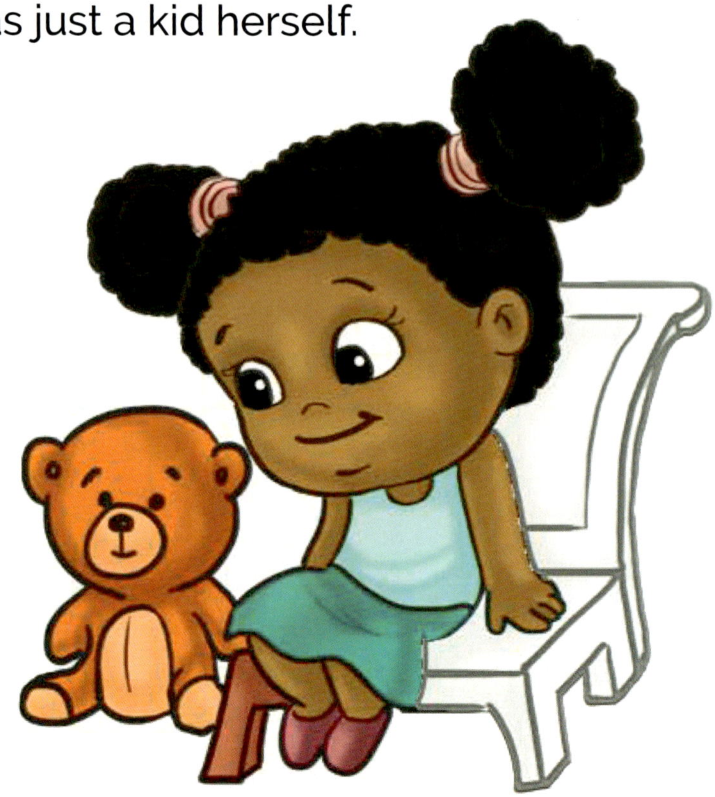

When Chuki and Aisha argued, Selma pictured Jamiyah sending each of them to a calm-down corner that was specially marked with their names.

Sometimes when she didn't want to deal with any of them at all, in her mind, Selma would instruct Jamiyah to hire a baby-sitter to manage the squabblers.

Then Jamiyah and she would kick back to take a well-deserved break.

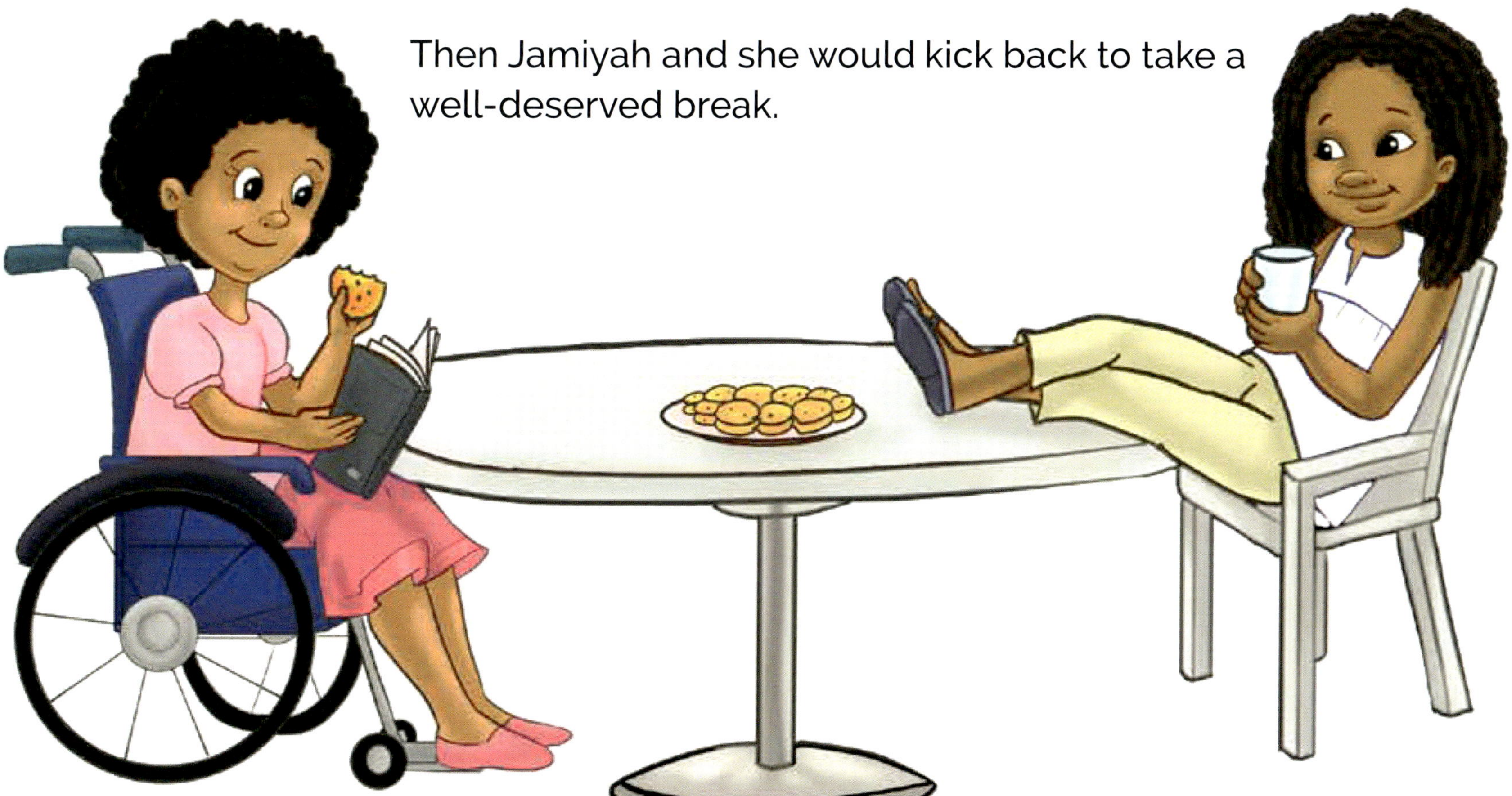

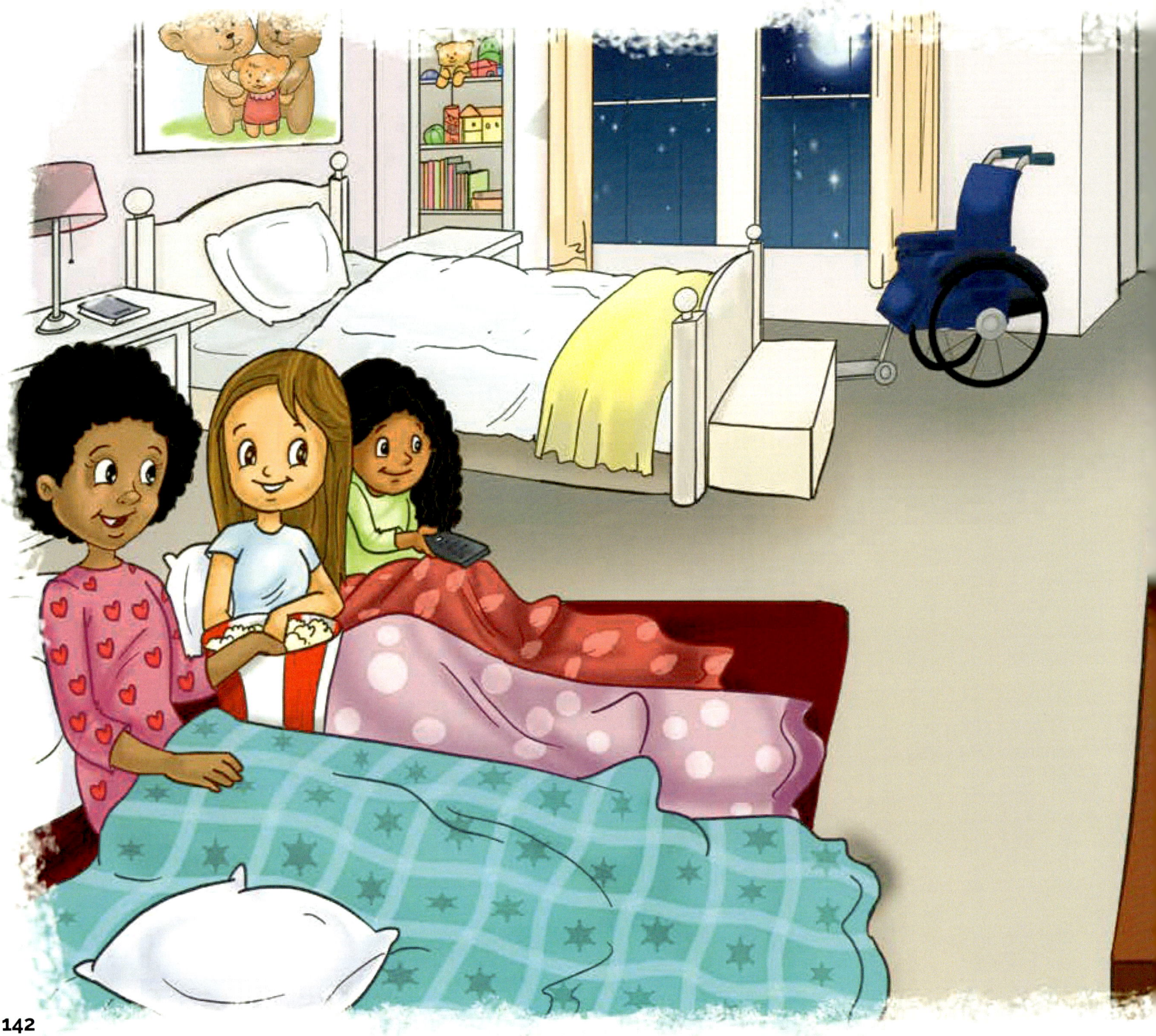

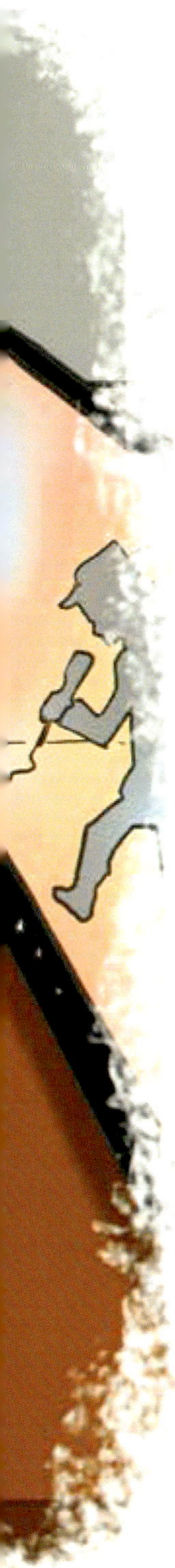

Not only did Selma's room become a smell-free and clutter-free zone, things at school and home got better.

And she started to participate more in social situations too!

VOILA!!!

Selma **felt better** about herself. She was able to successfully live with her voices.

Although she felt sad for her sisters, she no longer felt guilty or responsible for what her father had done to them.

Now that you have seen how Selma and Carlos managed their voices, I bet you're wondering what happened to Chang's Mr Charlie.

Chang came to discover that his grandparents and teachers were not right about his voice.

He really was not making up his voice or the noises. He really did hear them.

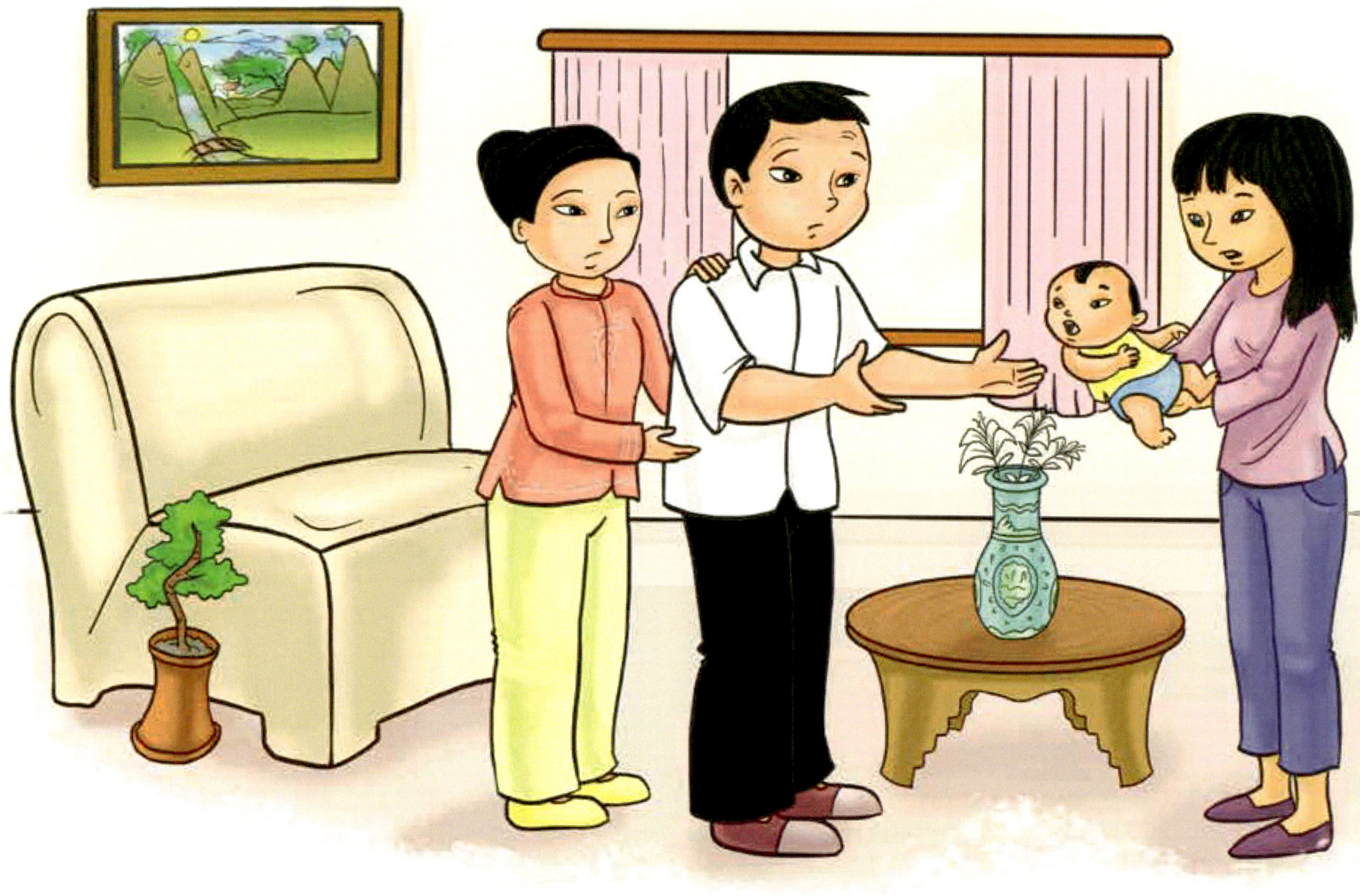

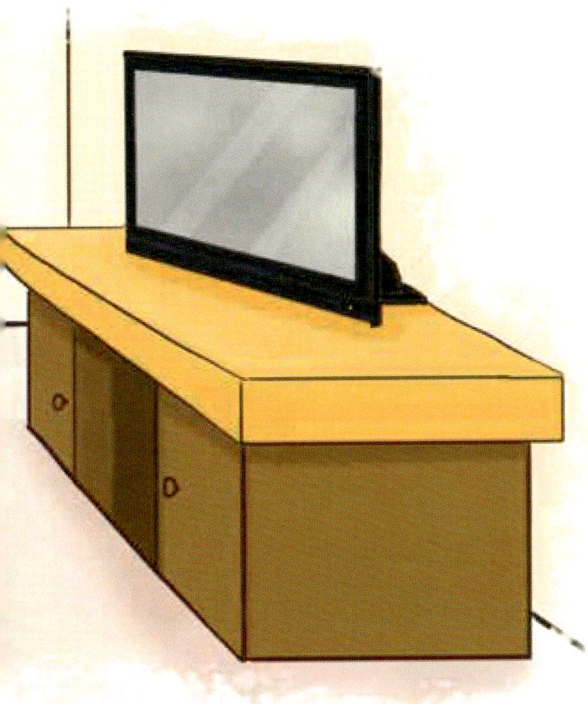

He also learned that the reason why he lived with his grandparents was because his mother was not able to take care of him. She suffered from a psychological condition called Schizophrenia that usually only adults have.

Part of the difficulty of living with Schizophrenia is that one hears voices, noises and sees things that are not there.

Chang's counselor told him that just because a family member hears voices does not mean that a kid will also hear voices when she's a child or when she becomes an adult. But it is possible.

Just because someone hears voices when he is a kid does not mean that he will definitely hear them when he becomes an adult. But it is possible.

One more thing Chang learned was that if an adult hears voices, their life is not ruined. Voices can be managed.

Hearing voices can be a part of life.

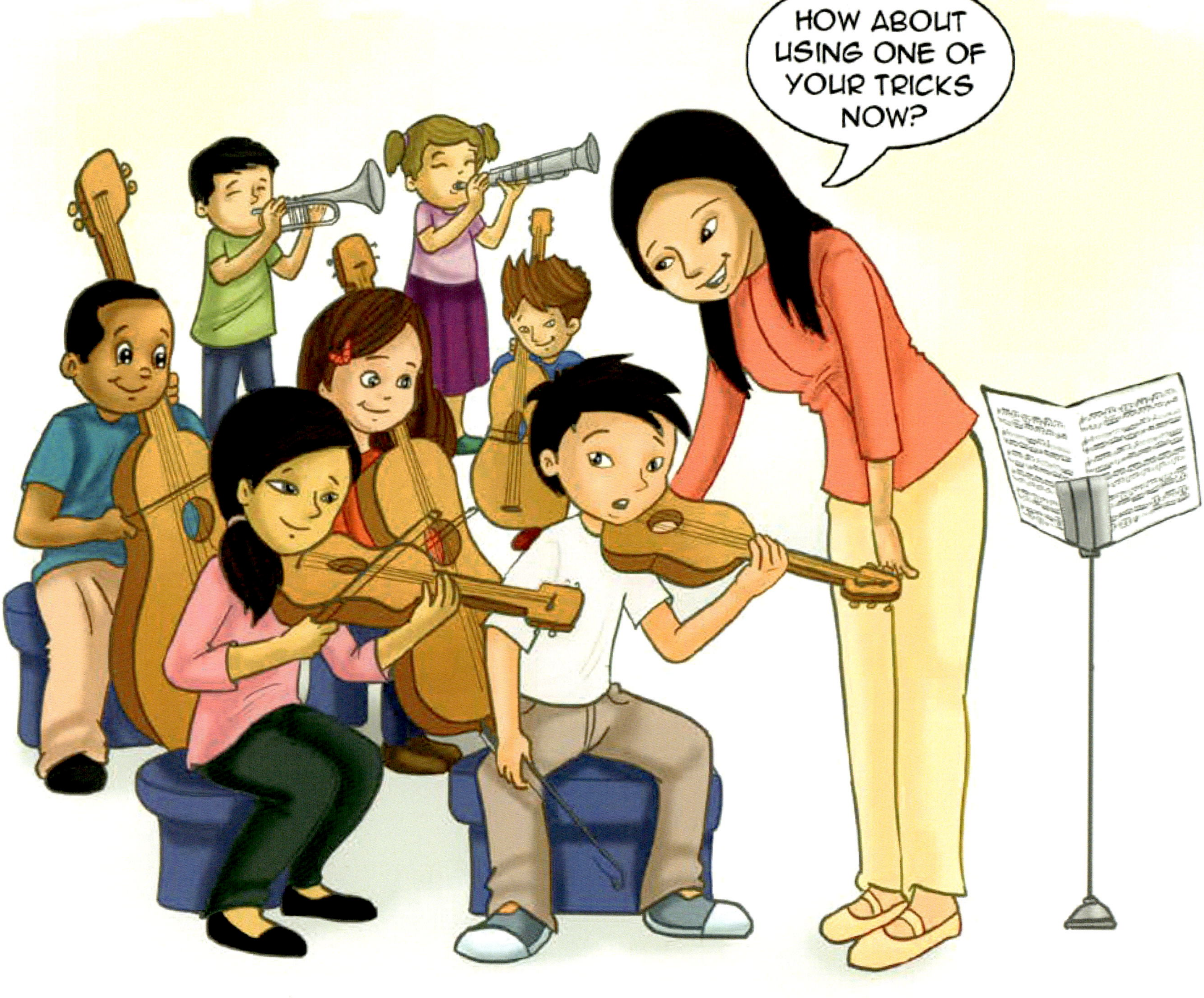
HOW ABOUT USING ONE OF YOUR TRICKS NOW?

Chang felt much better when he heard that he was not "making up" the noises he heard. He felt even more relieved to know it is possible to manage voices and live with them.

With his counselor's help, Chang discovered that the way one feels about, thinks of and responds to voices makes a difference in your life.

Chang noticed that when he started feeling less worried, angry and scared about the voices, he felt calmer and happier.

Once Chang's grandparents and schoolteachers understood what Chang was struggling with, they started to help him when they could.

When Chang looked like he was staring at "nothing" or seemed like he was preoccupied, they helped bring Chang's attention back to the classroom.

They said something like, "Chang, how about using one of your TRICKS now?" to remind him of the tricks that he had crafted to help himself manage his voices.

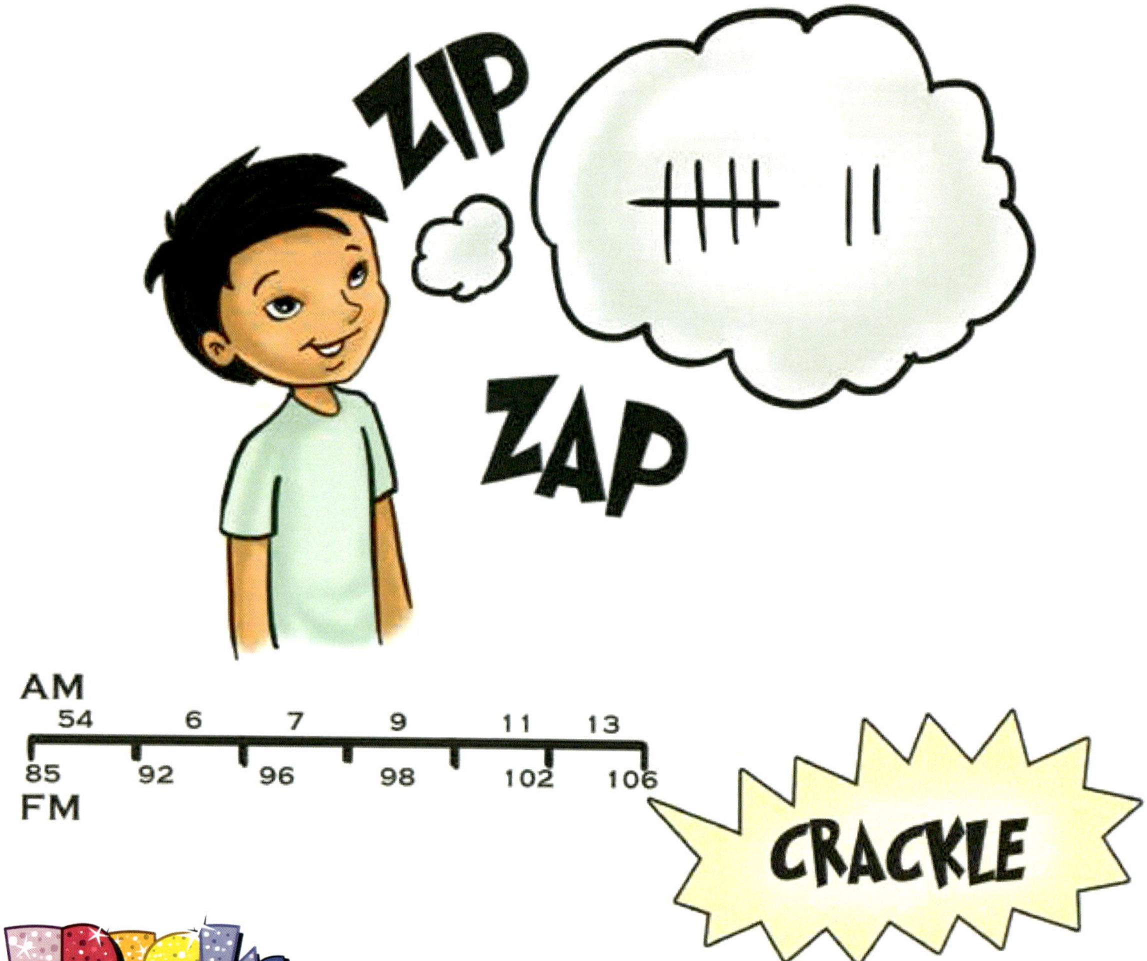

Some of the TRICKS Chang developed were:

(i) Saying "Stop!" to the voices and noises.

(ii) Making a mental note of the crackling noises by keeping count of their frequency.

(iii) Changing the "channel" from "static" to "easy listening."

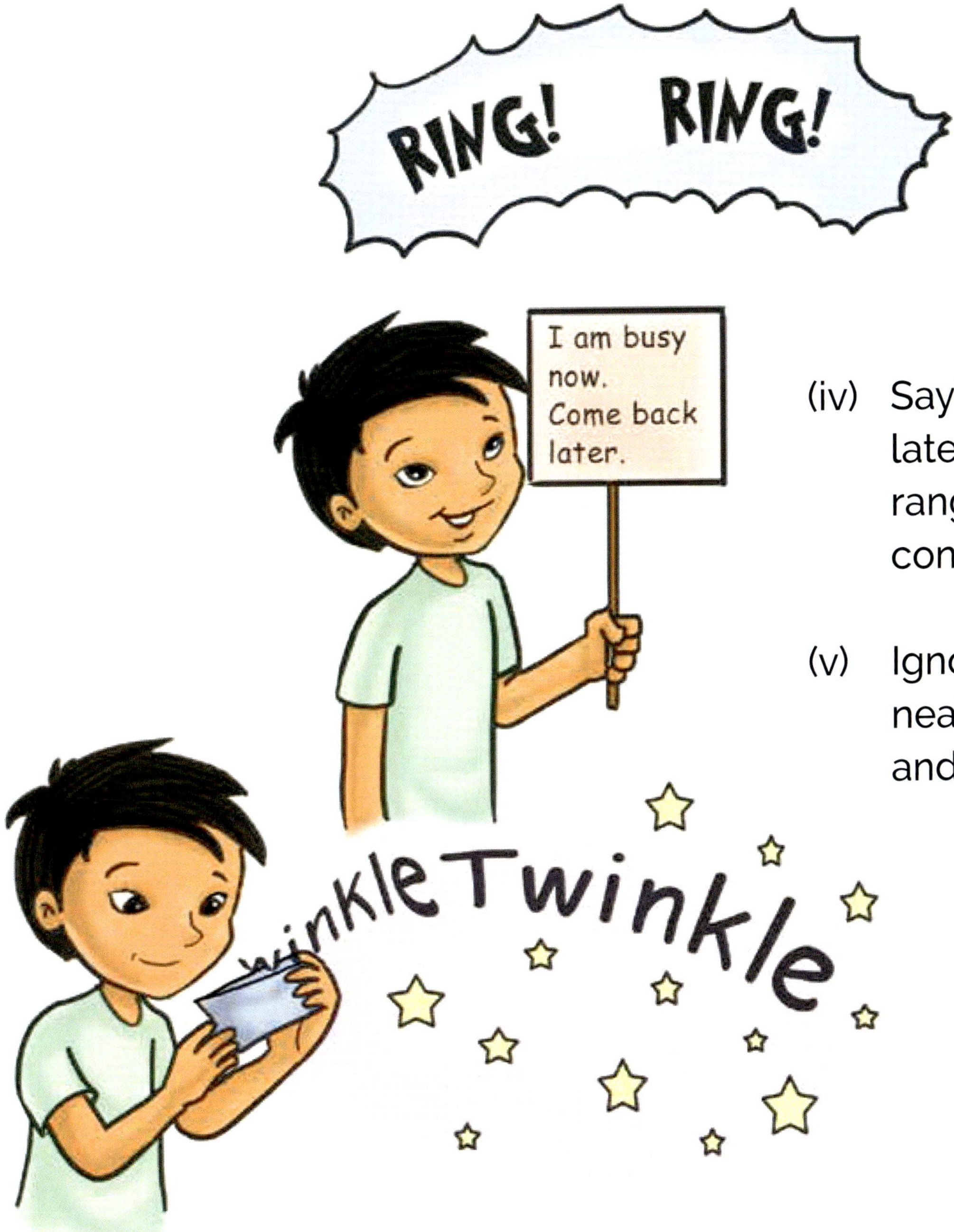

(iv) Saying "I'm busy now, come back later" if the phone or doorbell rang and he didn't feel like having a conversation.

(v) Ignoring Mr Charlie or imagining neatly putting him into an envelope and sealing it tight.

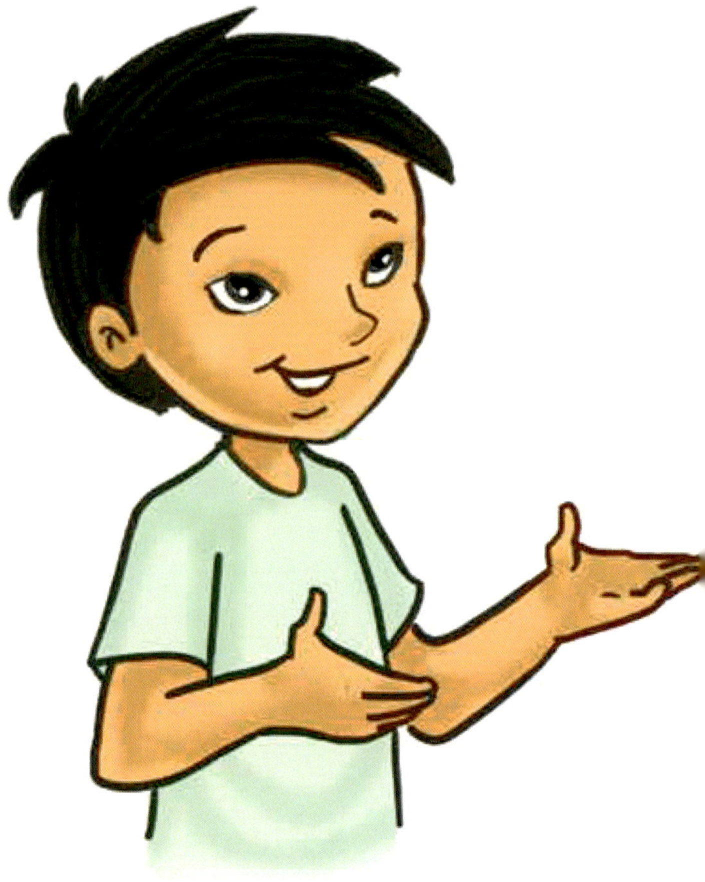

Chang got used to expecting Mr Charlie and the noises at any time. But he noticed something different in his life.

He explained to his counselor that "Voices and noises are things that my brain just does. It is neither 'bad' nor 'good'. It just 'is' and I always get to choose whether to entertain them and how I manage them."

Chang liked being in charge of his voices. He didn't find them so dreadful and bothersome anymore.

Slowly, Chang was better able to complete school assignments and chores at home. He also didn't need to eat as frequently to quieten Mr Charlie.

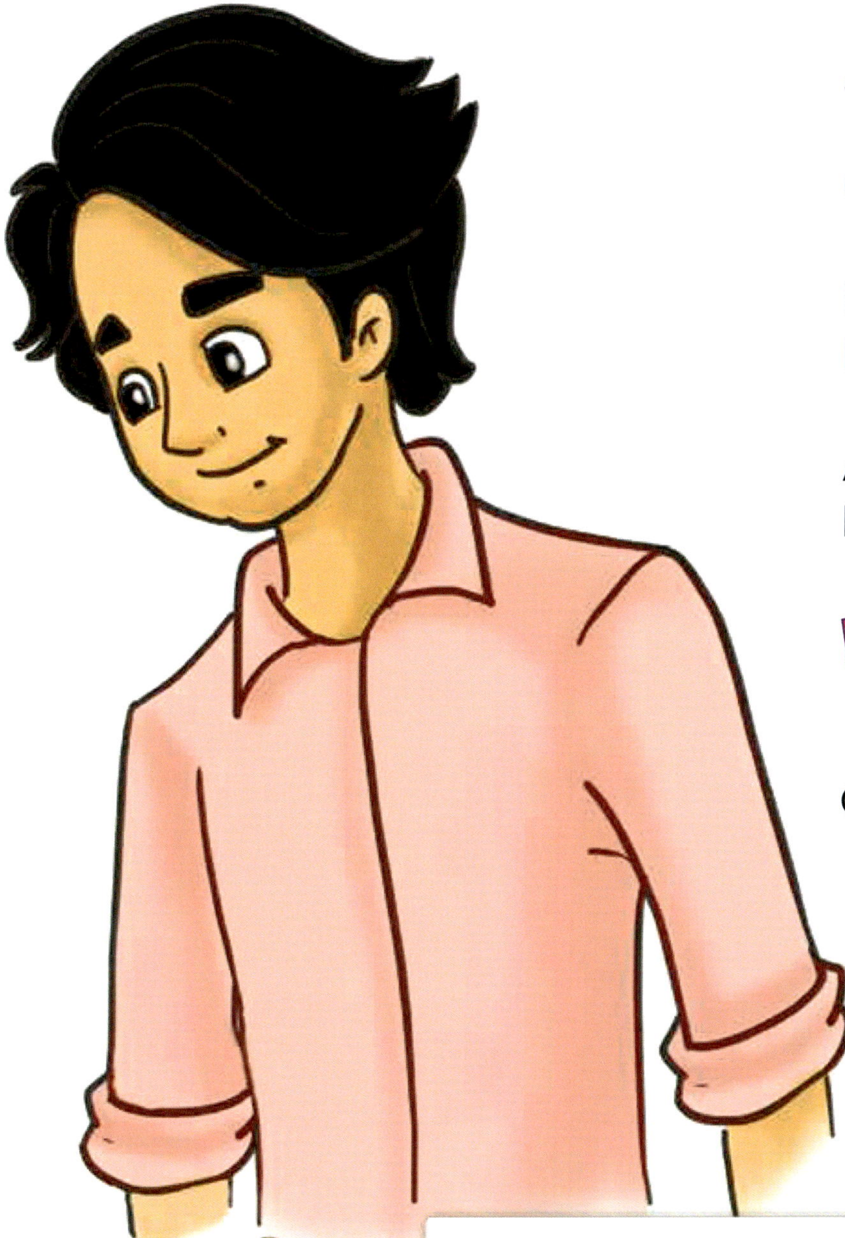

And guess what?

Chang also ended up losing weight!

His doctor and grandparents were very happy for him.

All in all, Chang **felt better** about himself and life felt good.

Hooray!!!

Chang learned to live with his voice!

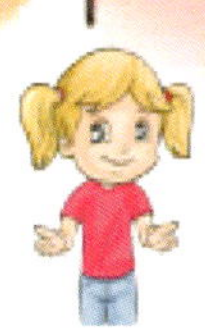

Are you curious to know what happened to La-la and whether she still misses her mommy? Go on to the next page to find out.

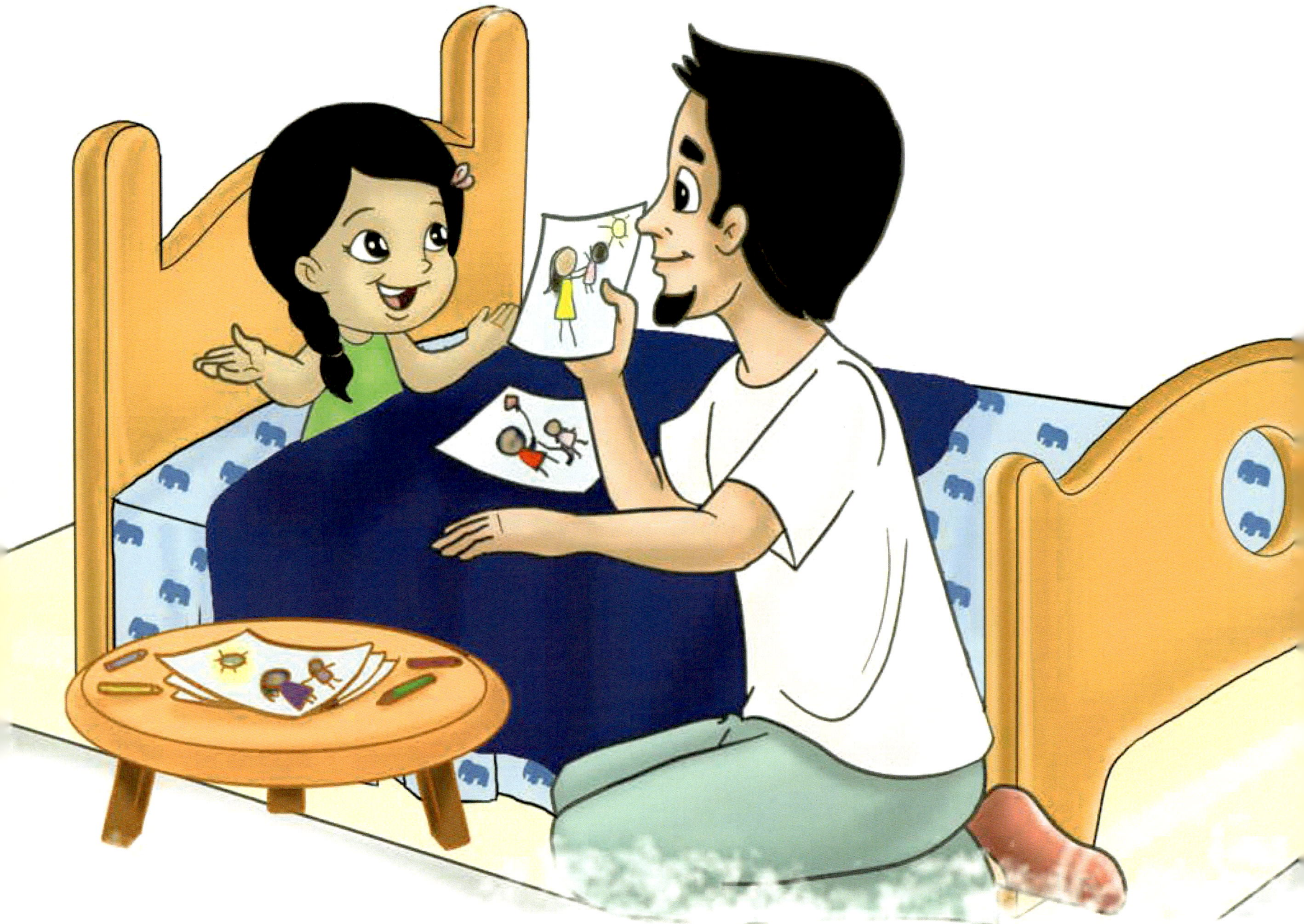

La-la learned that a lot of people find it hard to say goodbye to someone they love very much when they die.

It is normal to feel sad.

It is also common for people to think about or imagine their loved-one after they are gone. This helps them keep the memory of their loved-one alive in their minds.

Although La-la didn't really want to stop seeing or hearing her mom's voice, she did realize that her mom was no longer alive.

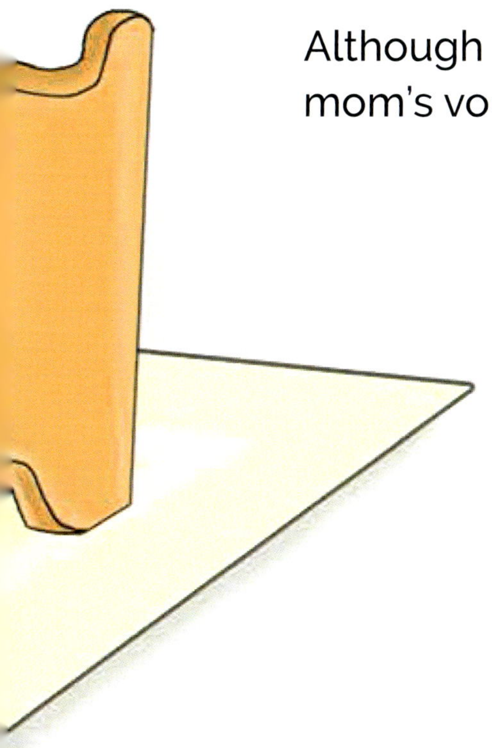

What helped La-la was drawing pictures of her mom and of the happy memories they had shared together.

La-la always had drawing paper, crayons and color pencils by her bed.

Every time she thought of her mom she would draw a picture about it. This way she wouldn't forget the memories. And she wouldn't have to keep them all in her head.

La-la shared all her drawings with her dad every day.

Six weeks later, La-la's mom's voice came and went now and then and no longer got in the way of her bedtime.

La-la still enjoyed going to bed.

She got to spend special father-and-daughter time with her dad. They talked and read stories together.

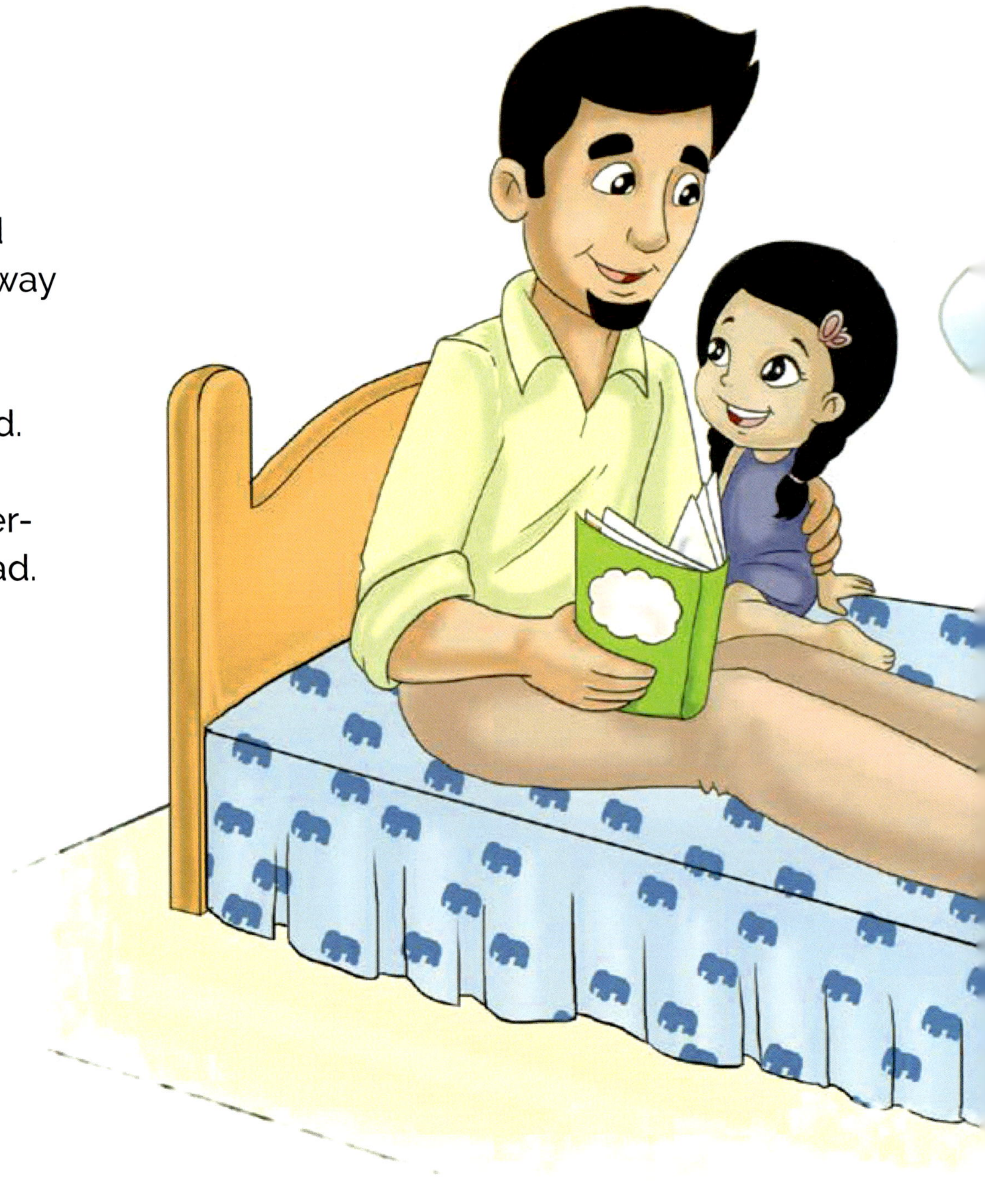

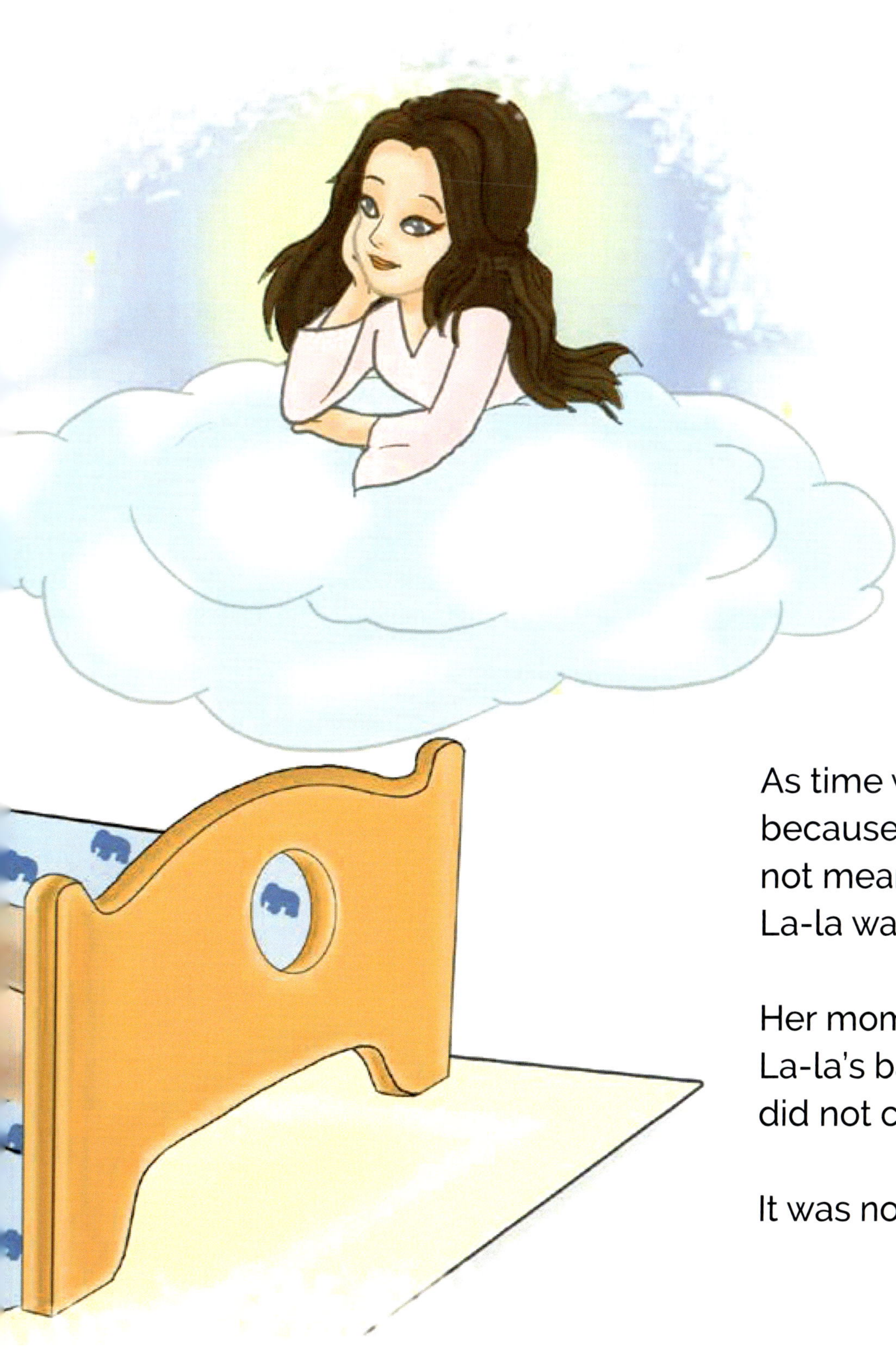

As time went on, La-la knew that just because her mom was not returning, did not mean that she did not love her or that La-la was unlovable.

Her mom did not go away because of La-la's bad behavior and La-la certainly did not cause her mom to go away.

It was not her fault.

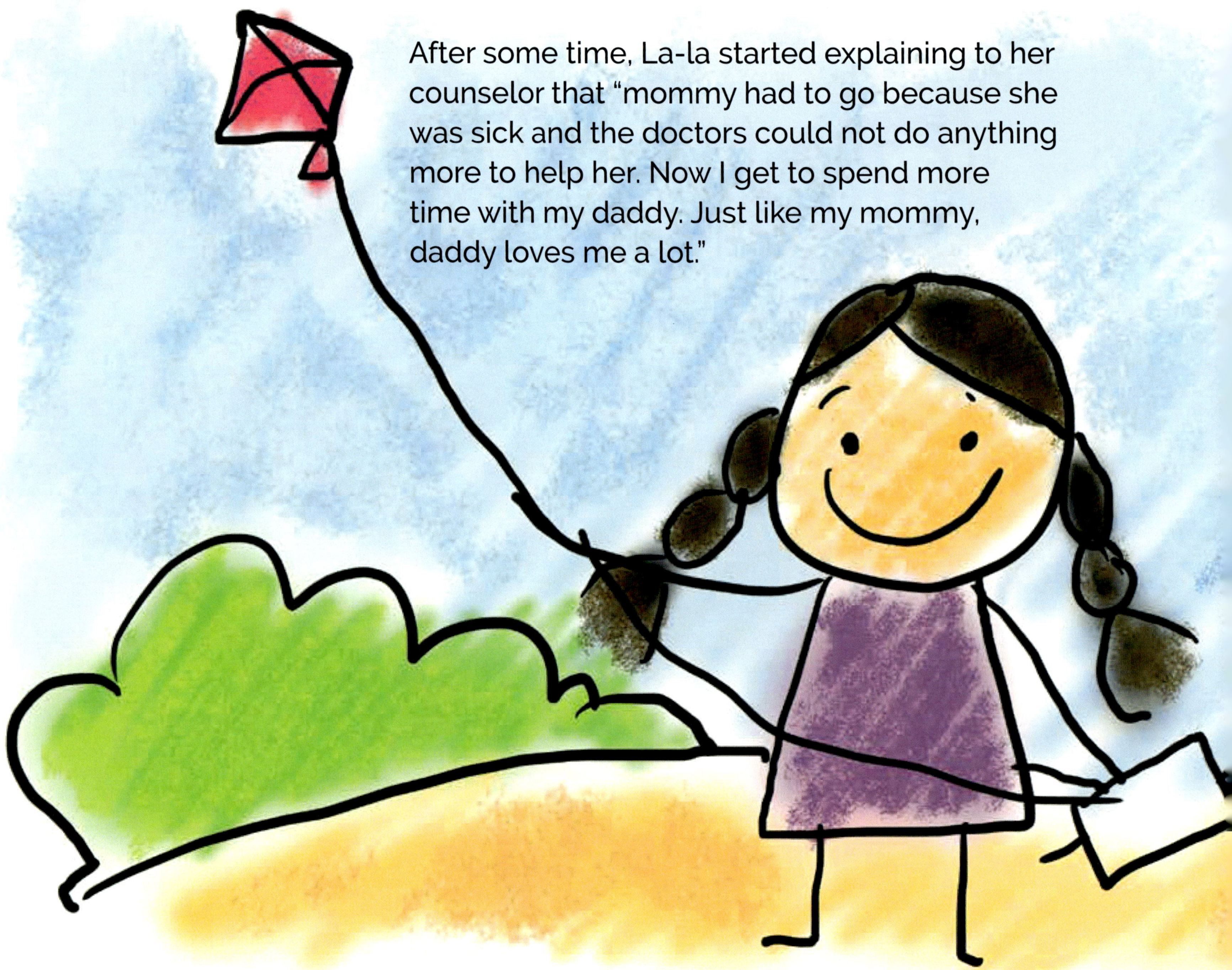

After some time, La-la started explaining to her counselor that "mommy had to go because she was sick and the doctors could not do anything more to help her. Now I get to spend more time with my daddy. Just like my mommy, daddy loves me a lot."

La-la has drawn a picture of how she feels now. Look at her drawing below.

What do you think she feels?

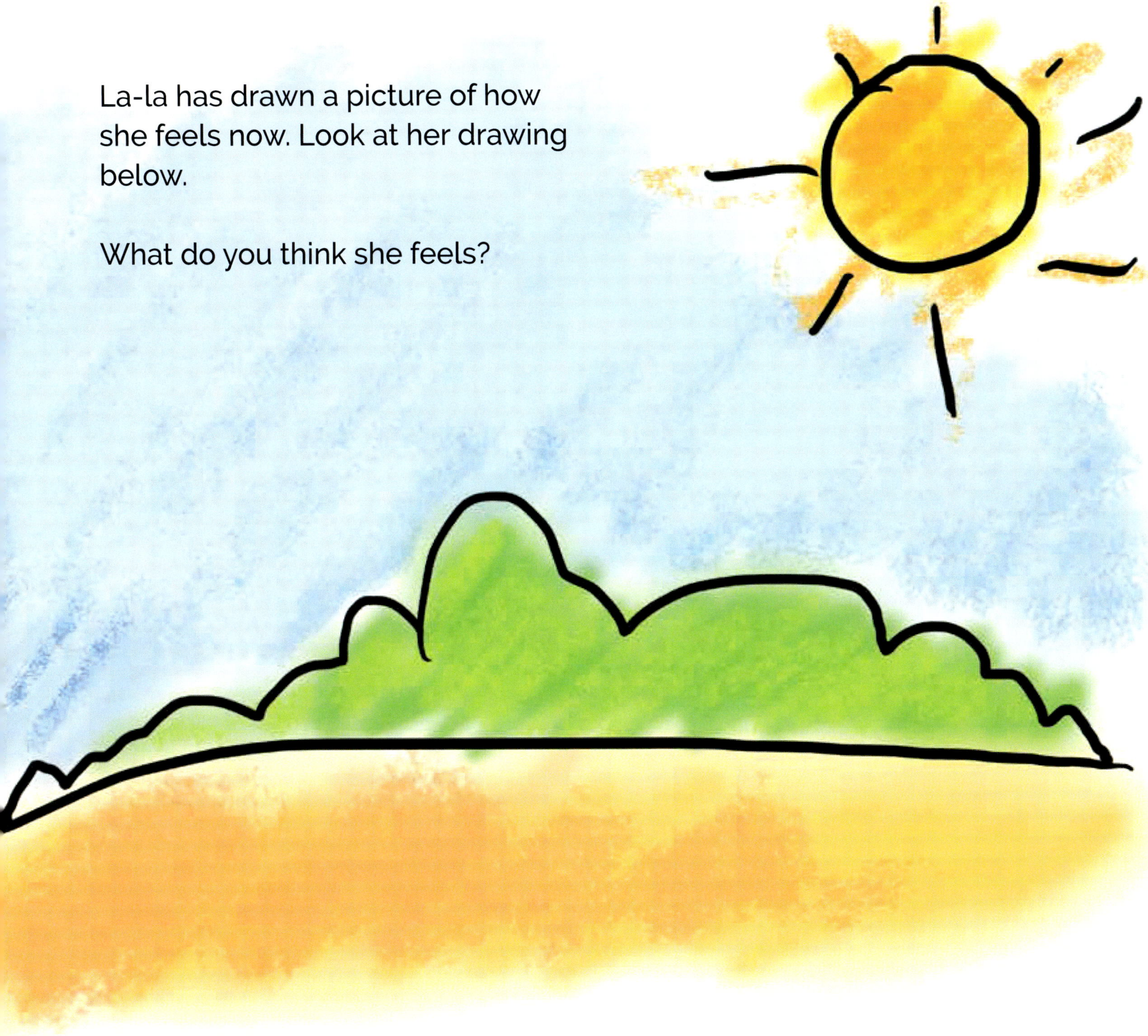

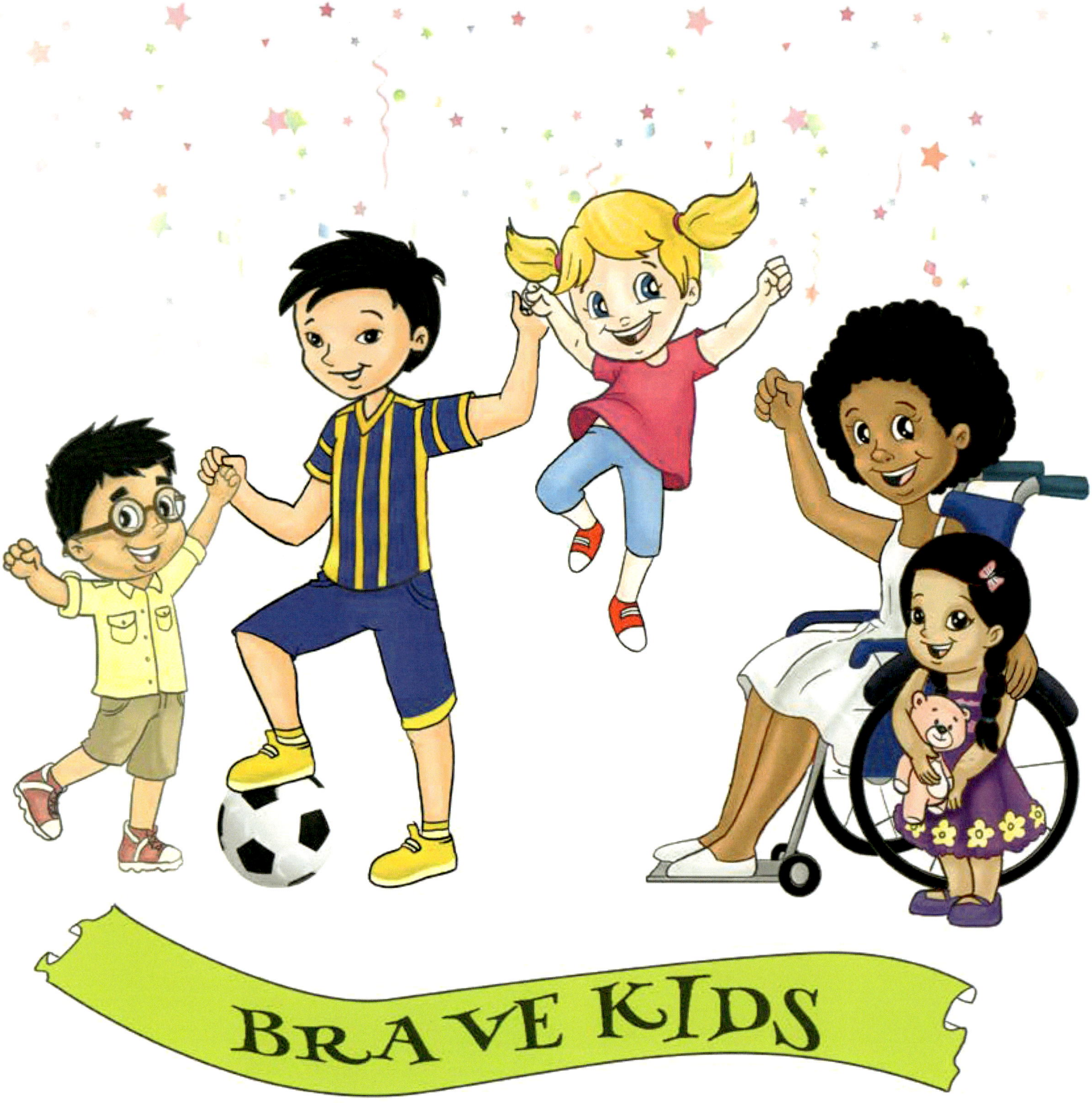
BRAVE KIDS

Would you like to understand and manage your voices like Carlos, Selma, Chang, La-la and me?

Speak to an adult you trust or a counselor to see if they can help you understand your voices. If talking to someone and using tricks don't help with managing the voices immediately, **don't give up**. There are other things that can help you.

Talk to a counselor and he or she will help you figure out how to manage your voices.

Don't forget, it takes a lot of **courage** to talk about voices.

It took each of us some time to learn about the role voices played in our lives and then how to cope with them. It was hard for all of us.

You're not alone. Just keep at it.

WE DID IT AND SO CAN YOU!

Wishing you all the best in your journey!

Susie, Carlos, Selma, Chang and La-la